# VET IN THE VALE

## *A Star Original*

'Well, fancy trying to castrate an old mare! Didn't they teach you anything at college?'

I seized the instruments from him and went back into the stygian gloom. We repeated the previous procedure, and managed to create three geldings. Paddy made a grab at the last, got the rope round its head, and I caught its tail as it jumped forward. But just at that moment, I tripped. Putting out my hand to save myself, I grabbed hold of a mane belonging to one of our earlier successes. He, feeling rightly indignant at a further assault on his dignity, hurled himself at the wall.

What happened next remains a blur. There was a loud crack and then a slow tearing sound. The stable was full of flying objects, and, looking back on it, I can imagine what it feels like to be caught in an earthquake. Jim swears that the stable distintegrated like a house of cards, and that when the dust settled, all that could be seen was my rear pointed skywards, and Paddy's cap in a heap of tile and wattle.

Also by David Dawson in *Star*

**VET IN DOWNLAND**

# VET IN THE VALE

David Dawson

*illustrated by*
Graham Allen

**A STAR BOOK**

Published by
the Paperback Division of
W. H. Allen & Co. Ltd

A Star Book
Published in 1978
by the Paperback Division of
W. H. Allen & Co. Ltd.
A Howard and Wyndham Company
44 Hill Street, London W1X 8LB

Printed in Great Britain by
C. Nicholls & Company Ltd.
The Philips Park Press, Manchester

ISBN 0 352 30209 7

# BOMBSHELL

AFTER I had been working in the veterinary practice for about five years, dealing with horses of all descriptions, I graduated to the exalted role of senior assistant. This meant that not only was there a junior vet, to whom even I could occasionally pass on the duller jobs, but also that I was allowed to regard a small number of the clients as my own responsibility. A mixed blessing for them, but for me an unmitigated joy. I watched over their brood like a mother hen, worrying unduly when one was sick and boasting shamelessly when one actually won a race. True, it was rarely more than a "seller", but, to listen to my ecstatic reports to Jim Enoch in the yard, it might have won a classic.

Among my flock at this time was an old man called George Makepeace, who, in his day, had been one of the leading National Hunt trainers and had won two Cheltenham Gold Cups. He was now in his seventies, and, rather than retire, kept himself occupied with about a dozen moderate jumpers. A lean, kindly, grey-haired gentleman of the old school, generous to a fault, but always immaculately turned out in a Saville Row tweed suit and shoes which were so highly polished they shone in the sun. Pernickety about his own comforts, he was the same with horses'. The boxes were in perfect order, and nothing but the very best forage was good enough for his charges. Their every whim was catered for, and, as a result, there were few days when I was not summoned to attend to some minor or even imaginary ailment at Letcombe Grange.

I had just got home one evening, when George phoned. "David," he said. "That bay gelding, Bombshell, who broke a blood vessel at Buckfastleigh last week, did the same again

5

this morning on the gallops. I know you listened to his heart and said he had a whistle in it and that he would probably never be reliable again. Well, I saw Gerald Wood at the races today and he told me that he has some marvellous new drug from America which I can try. It has to be injected intravenously one hour before the race, so could you come to Chepstow next Tuesday and give him a shot?'

Trying not to sound too enthusiastic, I replied that I thought I could manage to get away for the afternoon. I warned him that, like all the other miracle cures for blood-vessel breakers, this one had no guarantee. In fact, I knew of this new potion, which was a dilute acid with supposed ability to encourage the blood to clot with great rapidity in the lungs. I had heard one of the partners discussing this drug. It appeared that two horses had been given an injection and had raced uneventfully. Because of this, the drug was hailed as a miracle cure round the racecourses. But the chief problem with this condition is its unpredictability. A horse may bleed in one race and then run two without, only to bleed again during a canter on the home gallops.

However, I arranged to meet George the following Tuesday, and proudly announced in the surgery that I would be away that afternoon at Chepstow. Not unexpectedly, this was greeted with considerable ridicule.

"You'll be the only one off, then," was Jim's comment.

"You must have guessed that I'd arranged for you to do all the horse's teeth at Beckhampton that day," said Mr Grill, with a grin.

The Captain looked up from the table, where he was rolling one of his herbal smoke canisters, "You'd better watch out," he growled. "If you're seen walking round the racecourse with a hypodermic syringe, they'll have you in before the stewards quicker than lightning."

"Good God!" I spluttered. "It's not illegal to inject a horse before racing, is it?"

"Well not exactly illegal, but damned unsporting. If the Press boys get to hear of it, they'll really go to town."

I could see it all – *Vet Caught Doping Horse*. What a

headline in Wednesday's *Sporting Life*. Next stop would be the Disciplinary Committee of the Royal College of Veterinary Surgeons. "No Dawson, disgraceful conduct, barred from practice for one year." I could hear the verdict being pronounced. "I think I'll ring George to say I can't get off on Tuesday," I said, as I saw my hand beginning to twitch.

"Oh, go on, David. Can't you see the Captain is wildly envious of your day's racing," laughed Eric. "Of course it's not illegal, although I don't think they'll allow it much longer. You go off and enjoy yourself. You'll have enough worries keeping George out of the bar without bothering about the stipendiary stewards."

Tuesday duly arrived, bringing another damp, cold south-westerly wind driving across the Downs. I made an early start and managed to complete my morning calls by mid-day. Driving into the yard to collect my racing clothes and glasses, I was met by Billy Foster, the new assistant. He rushed up to the car as I pulled up. "Hurry up, David. The Press Association have sent a man down to interview you about Bombshell's chances this afternoon ... He wants to come with you and take some pictures of you treating the horse."

I was appalled. How on earth had they found out? Surely it must be a leg-pull. "Billy, don't be such an idiot. Do grow up and remember that you're no longer a student," I answered irritably. I knew that my colleague was an habitual practical joker; a habit which we all suspected he had acquired through being born in a police car in Buenos Aires, where his father had been British Consul.

"No, it's quite genuine," he replied. "He's in the office with Jim Enoch. His name's Percy Dalkeith. He's been waiting for an hour already."

Stunned by this news, I made my way into the office, wondering how on earth he had found out and how I could possibly get rid of him. I could still back out and make some excuse that an urgent case had cropped up, leaving me no time to get to Chepstow. But Bombshell was in the second last race, and according to the newspapers was favourite, so obviously George Makepeace fancied his chances. I could not let George down. Perhaps I could stop for petrol on the way, somehow contrive to get my companion out of the car and then drive off without him.

Turning these and other dire possibilities over in my mind, I went in to be confronted by Jim, wearing his most puckish of grins, and a tall, lean figure in a well-fitting check suit. "Hello, David, my boy. You've cut it pretty fine. This is Mr Dalkeith from the P.A. .... He wants to have a few words with you and grab a lift to the races."

"Pleased to meet you, Mr Dawson," the tall man drawled. "Mr Enoch has been telling me all about this new wonder drug, which you have brought over from the States. He tells me it's expected to transform this horse today. My office have just rung to tell me that there are thousands of pounds going on him all over the country. It'll be a great scoop for me to have the exclusive story and pictures."

"Really, Mr Dalkeith, I'm sure that there has been some mistake. I have no intention of doing anything dramatic to Bombshell. In fact, I don't believe that my presence will make any difference to his performance. I'm sure that you are wasting your time and that somebody has fed you wrong information."

"Not at all, David. May I call you David, by the way?"

Weakly I nodded assent.

"Not at all. You are too modest. But you'd better change or we'll be late. I can ask you some questions as we drive there."

"Quite right, Percy, old boy," said Jim, hovering over me and holding my suit and rather battered hat. 'You can get the whole story from him in the car. We are all very proud of him today, to say nothing of the fact that we're going to make a lot of money."

Before I could make any further protest, I found myself changed and bundled into the driving seat with the ever-present Percy alongside me. I started the engine and let in the clutch just as Jim stuck his head through the car window.

Looking more evil than usual, he palmed a parcel into my hand. "What the hell is this?" I said, getting more and more irritable.

"Don't forget the medicine," he said in a stage whisper. My God, in my consternation I had completely forgotten about it. Taking it, I drove off as Jim wished us luck and Percy a good story. I had the impression that he winked conspiratorially at my companion, but I was too flustered to be sure. I still had no inkling of an idea as to how I was to lose my passenger, and I cursed myself for having mentioned the whole ridiculous matter in the surgery. I could easily have gone off without telling anyone until the last moment, but, as usual, my feelings of importance at being asked to go to treat a horse at the races had carried me away. I told Dalkeith that we would have to drive fast as we were half an hour behind schedule, and set off towards Gloucester like Stirling Moss. Perhaps he would take fright and jump out. At any rate, the speed seemed to depress his powers of conversation.

Passing Cirencester, the road straightened out for Gloucester, and Percy took his courage in his hands.

"Now tell me about this drug," he began. "Will it really make this old horse run a stone better than he has before?"

My blood ran cold. What on earth had they been telling him? I began to explain the whole medical condition of Epistaxis (blood-vessel bleeding), using as many scientific terms as I could rake up from the depths of my memory. So long as I kept talking about veterinary science, I could keep him off his insinuations of doping and large gambles. By the time my ideas had run dry, we had gone through Gloucester and were heading down the Chepstow road.

"I think we can slow down a bit now," my companion volunteered. "We've still got more than an hour to the first race."

Assuring him that speed was essential, I continued to throw the car round the twisting bends of the Wye valley as though the devil himself was after us. As we neared Chepstow I began to slow down, and Percy started to breathe at a more normal speed. "Jesus, do you vets always drive like that?" he queried.

"Only when we're under stress," I replied. "I'm sure that you don't want to be late if you've got copy to write on the first race."

Percy looked across and said that actually he was only interested in the fifth race and so we had plenty of time.

As we pulled into the trainers' car park, Percy coughed and asked rather apologetically if I could get him a pass into the Members'.

"But surely you have a press badge for all courses?" I asked.

"Well, actually, old boy, I'm afraid there's been a bit of a con job. You see I'm not really a press man. In fact, I'm Billy Foster's uncle. I was visiting him for the weekend, and he persuaded me to stay on and come racing. He and Jim Enoch thought up this story to persuade you to take me to the races. If I'd known how badly you drive I'd have gone straight home."

"You bastard," I said grinning with relief. "It serves you damn well right. I only drove like that to frighten you from asking stupid questions. Well, now you are here, I'll try and get you in. But that's more than I'll do for your blasted nephew when I get home."

Followed by Percy, I made my way to the Owners' and Trainers' gate, gave my name to the official and said that I was working for Mr Makepeace. The gatekeeper acknowledged me and handed me a pass. "Could you possibly let me have another pass for my friend here? His name's Dalkeith and he is a leading Australian racing journalist. He would very much like to meet his English colleagues."

The man was most helpful and said that not only would he see that my friend had a pass, but he would personally arrange for him to be introduced to the members of the press box. So, leaving Percy speechless in the hands of the official, I made my escape to meet George in the Members' bar.

I found George with his owner, a Derbyshire steel man, busy priming themselves for the day's activities on vodka and tonics. Buying me a drink, George inquired whether I was in good order and had brought the necessary materials. I assured him that all was well, and asked whether he fancied Bombshell's chances.

"Well he is and good his chance," replied the owner, who appeared throughout the day to talk in this rather prosaic form of English.

"So long as the medicine works, he should run well," said George. "He has better form than the other five runners, if only he runs as I know he can. Still, I don't think we can risk a big bet on him. I've told Charlie here not to have more than a monkey on him." Hoping that £500 did not count as a big bet, I took it that no great gamble was anticipated. "I'll meet you at the stables after the third race," said George. "I've told the veterinary officer what we are doing and he is quite happy."

Heartened by the news that I was not breaking every rule of racing, I set off to see the first two races. I had a modest investment of fifty pounds on an old selling hurdler of Bill Carver's from Lambourn, whom I had had to stitch up a month ago when he misjudged a schooling hurdle on Mann Down. I figured that this misadventure might have made him more careful in the future. He duly won by several lengths, having jumped like a buck, at the noble odds of ten to one. As I walked past the unsaddling enclosure, I was delighted to see my companion Percy surrounded by press boys, and obviously discomforted by their questions. Serve him right, I thought. I hope they give him a real grilling on the Melbourne Cup.

The third race finished and I made my way to the race-course stables, clutching my syringe and bottle in my trouser pocket. I felt like a tourist trying to smuggle an extra packet of cigarettes through customs. I met George at the gate, and he led me uneventfully through to the box where Bombshell was being brushed over by his lad. The gelding allowed me to insert the needle into his vein and administer the agreed dose without a protest. I quickly went back to my car and disposed of the evidence in the boot. When I returned to

11

the course, the horses for the chase were parading in the first ring. The remainder looked to be of not very high class. Three had been fired, one was clearly living in a hotel where the food was not all it might be and the other was a big raw-boned grey with "cat-hairs" missed by the clippers.

In the paddock I joined George and the owner. "Quiet as you ride and steady he will run. Drive as you can from the last and win he will," the owner told the jockey, in his strange monosyllabic way. The jockey muttered some toothless comment about the bugger winning if he jumped, and clambered aboard ready to head for the start. Climbing to the top of the stands, I waited for the starter to call them into line.

What do I say if he pulls up with a broken blood vessel? I thought. Poor George is quite convinced that this is a wonder drug.

I looked out over the superb panorama of Chepstow, which has since become one of my favourite racecourses. The big, ambitiously designed track is situated in four hundred acres of glorious parkland where the Wye Valley runs in to the Severn estuary, the green grass and gay racing colours sensationally set off by the vividly contrasting backdrop of dark trees and rugged grey cliffs that border the great salmon river. It is left-handed and caters for jumping and flat-racing. About two miles round, it undulates sharply and the switchback straight seems to appeal to most horses. But, I thought ominously, you need a horse with plenty of stamina to win if the going is at all heavy, as it was that day. And I had a feeling that Bombshell was a little short of this commodity. We would soon know the answer.

The small field set off at a respectable pace for the first circuit. As they came past the stands first time round, Bombshell was pulling his jockey's arms out in second place behind a big brown horse with heavily fired legs. At the end of the back straight, the grey shot into the lead with our hope still lying second or third. The grey was two lengths clear at the second last, where the brown horse tripped up, leaving

12

Bombshell as the only serious danger. Suddenly he slowed almost to a walk, and over the last, the three horses behind him all jumped past. At the finish the grey horse was ten lengths clear and we were a distant fifth. I came down from the stands and joined a disconsolate group standing around Bombshell outside the unsaddling enclosure.

"Farther he went, slower he ran," barked the owner, making off for the bar.

"Did he break?" I asked George.

"Not so far, David. See what he's like in the stables in half an hour. The jockey said he was interfered with at the last," George said happily enough. This seemed strange in that he had apparently stopped well before the last, but at least it seemed that the drug had worked, and the old trainer had a satisfactory explanation before following to the bar.

While the horses paraded for the last race I made my way to the stables. I found Bombshell quietly standing in his box, quite unperturbed by his day out.

"No sign of any blood?" I asked his lad.

He assured me that he had not seen a trace, and that the old horse was a real villain and would not do a tap more than he wanted. That seemed to be that. So I turned on my heel and made for the exit. On the way, I passed a box where four or five men were excitedly talking in Welsh. Looking in as I passed, I saw the grey victor standing in the centre of the box with blood pouring from both nostrils. "Can I help?" I volunteered. "I am a vet."

"No, lad," replied a large florid Welshman, who appeared to be the trainer. "He always does this, helps to clear the bad blood from him. Never any good he isn't unless he has a good bleed at the races."

Thoroughly chastened, I made my way back to report to George that all was well with Bombshell, and to suggest that next time he might let him run without an injection. As I walked to the weighing room, I was joined by Percy in a subdued mood. "Deuced hard day," he said lugubriously. "Bastards kept asking questions about some place called Wagga Wagga, said I must have heard of it. When I did escape from them, it was only to lose twenty-five quid for Jim, Billy and myself."

I did not feel particularly charitable towards that triumvirate, but at least we drove home at a more reasonable pace. As I arrived back at the surgery, I made a mental vow never to communicate my missions to the practice in the future.

# THE RAINSTORM

Jim and I were studying the day's runners in *Sporting Life* when Billy Foster burst through the surgery door. "Bother your clients, David. You're welcome to them." He sounded peeved and irritable. The latter I could understand, since I fully shared that emotion. We had been celebrating the Captain's farewell party until an early hour that morning, and none of us were too strong in the head.

"What on earth are you talking about? And for heaven's sake don't make such a noise," I grumbled, pushing the paper over to Jim. "Let's all have a cup of strong coffee. You can simmer down, and Jim can find out if that colt from Upper Lambourn really is fancied at Brighton today."

Jim shuffled off into the office to put the kettle on and to telephone one of his numerous relations, who was secretary to the trainer of our selected winner.

"Now then, Billy. What has upset your happy day?" I asked.

It seemed that Billy had been quietly making his way back from an early morning cattle job in Compton, when he had been stopped by one of Jack Melling's lads in Ilsley. Apparently one of their horses had got loose during first lot, and had gone berserk on the way home.

I asked which horse it was and learnt to my horror that it was a big black, called Rainstorm.

"He bloody well should have been called Brainstorm. It would have been more fitting. He's a ruddy savage," Billy retorted with much feeling.

Master Rainstorm was well known to me from past brushes. A powerful four-year-old colt, he had a considerable mind of his own, and, worse still, the strength to get his own way. On one occasion he had chased three of us out of

15

the box when I had been trying to dose him with a worm draught through a stomach tube. I had not particularly blamed him for objecting to this undignified form of treatment, but I had never forgiven him for grabbing hold of my favourite stomach tube and biting it in two halves.

As Jim returned with the coffee, I gradually pieced together the story of Billy's affray at Melling's. The string had been returning down the lane to the stable, when Rainstorm had arrived, breathless and furious from the gallops, where he had violently deposited and abandoned his rider. He had chased two of the fillies and then tried to remove a large slice of backside from one of the other colts. Being thwarted from the object of his pleasure by the terror-stricken lad, he had fallen into the ditch and then staggered around until he collapsed in a thrashing heap at the side of the lane. Billy had arrived to survey the scene, wincing at each shout from the assembled stable staff. Forced into a diagnosis, he had plumped for a brain haemorrhage, and had injected, with considerable difficulty, a shot of morphia. Despite all their efforts, the horse had been unable to rise. So the shaken Billy had left them with instructions to watch him and report progress.

I was halfway through my coffee when the phone rang. It was Mr Melling. "Is that you David? You'd better come out straight away. I've got a horse on the ground in the middle of the lane, and I can't get my second lot out with him in the way. That young chap of yours has looked at him and given him an injection, but he seems to have made the animal worse."

I told Jack that I would be over straight away, put down the phone and cursed Billy for landing me in what seemed likely to be a rough job, just when I felt like creeping home to bed.

As I made my way out of the surgery, Jim shouted after me that Doris had said the colt was fancied so long as it was drawn within five of the rails, and that there were fourteen runners. Telling him to put me on a pound when he knew the draw, I drove off to the dreaded Rainstorm. Jack Melling

16

had sounded both cross and worried on the telephone. He was a man of vast experience with horses, and, if he was worried, I knew that the colt was in obvious trouble. I had been told by the lads that Rainstorm had only been kept in training that year with a view to winning the Ascot Gold Cup. Since it was only ten days away, it seemed that his year was going to be wasted. I drove over the Downs trying to work out what could have gone wrong with him. I could see no reason why he should suddenly have had a blood-vessel break in his brain simply from getting loose on the gallops. But then, of course, he had always been a bit cranky. Perhaps he had been developing a brain tumour, which had reached its peak, causing him to lose his senses. My mind raced desperately over those odd conditions which are chronicled in the recesses of the old veterinary books. The "blind staggers" was an illness which featured prominently in the pages. Embellished with engravings of wide-eyed horses plunging in the shafts of a cart, various authorities had explained that this was a sudden attack, invariably fatal unless relieved by immediate and copious drawing of blood. That fool Billy should have stuck a large needle into his vein and let off four or five pints. If only he had, I could still be nursing my hang-over in the quiet of the lovely Miss Bailey's kitchen, where even now I was due to give her over-fat show hack its monthly dose of vitamins.

There were two lanes down to the Ilsley stables. I chose the second, reasoning that the first one would bring me immediately face to face with my patient. I decided to put off the actual moment of encounter for as long as possible in the hope that nature would decide on a cure first. Turning the corner, I was met by the head lad. "My God, sir, you don't look too clever today," he said helpfully. "I thought I looked bad when I got in just now from that brute, but I look a king beside you."

"Is he up yet, Gerry?" I asked, more in hope than expectation.

"Not likely. He seems to be getting worse every minute. He's flinging his feet in all directions, trying to get up and

17

then tumbling over again. Watch out for his head when you touch him. He's tried to bite poor old Joe three times."

Well, bless Gerry for his faith. He at least was sure that I would get close enough to risk getting bitten. I was not.

I followed my guide up the lane to a point where I could see three or four people gathered round a horse. As I arrived they respectfully stood back a pace to let the principal within range of his patient. Hastening to encourage Joe to hold his head again, I went to pat the unfortunate colt's neck. His immediate reaction to this well-meant endearment was to slash at my hand with his teeth, and then to go into a galloping action with all four feet, making me jump rapidly onto the bank. Carefully I approached again, this time from behind. I covered his uppermost eye with my hand and sought out his pulse, where the artery ran under his lower jaw. That at least was strong and beating at a steady rate.

"Well, he isn't going to die yet," I said, trying to sound reassuring.

"Never mind about dying. How are you going to move him off my damned lane?" growled the trainer, who had just arrived back on the scene.

"Oh, Jack, don't be so beastly. We should get an ambulance for him." The voice of a young lady rose to a nearly hysterical squeak. I looked up – and there was the most ravishing red-head, on the brink of tears.

"I don't suppose you know the Contessa di Seraglia, do you, Dawson? She is the owner of this black peril."

Sensing that a foreign countess was more likely to have faith in my healing powers than my more down-to-earth English acquaintances, I felt confidence well up inside me. "Now never you mind, we'll have him up and well in no time," I smiled encouragingly.

I told Joe to pull on the reins, and, with my shoulder under the horse's, we hoisted him into a sitting position. Advising the spectators to clear the decks, I gave Rainstorm a mighty slap on his rump. He let out a roar, and plunged forward on his front legs, dragging his rear along the ground. Fearing that he had broken his back and was para-

18

lysed in his hind-quarters, I felt in my pocket for a safety pin. I tentatively pricked him along his back and down his hind legs. Far from losing sensitivity, he took the greatest exception to this, and lunged forwards once more. This time he lost balance and toppled over onto his other side.

"It's so cruel. I can't watch this beastly man hurting my poor horse," sobbed the countess as she turned towards the house. "That's better," Mr Melling sighed. "Now she's gone, we can all get under and lift him up."

"Hold on a minute," I warned. I had just noticed a couple of large swellings alongside his quarters on which he had been lying. I felt down them and found that there was firm enlargement in the skin over an area about the size of a soup plate. I stood back and looked up the lane.

"Where exactly did he fall in the ditch?" I asked Joe.

"Just below that gate post. I remember, because I thought he was going to catch my leg under the gate when he fell." I walked back to the spot. There in the bottom of the ditch was a large clump of nettles, which had been flattened by the horse's fall. So that was it. Simple enough when the penny dropped, but so simple, that it had never occurred to me before. Nettle stings do strange things to horses, one of which is to paralyse the hind-quarters. Suddenly optimistic and infinitely more cheerful, I told Joe to keep hold of Rainstorm, while I collected a syringe from the car. I assured Jack Melling that I would have his horse up before the second lot were due to come up the track.

I knew I had a bottle of an anti-histamine drug, which had been given to me on trial by one of the drug companies. I only hoped that I had remembered to put it in the car. It was said to have a dramatic effect on all varieties of allergic reactions. Scrabbling about on the back seat I found the bottle, re-read the instructions and filled a syringe. Going back to the horse, I had the impression that he was a lot more settled and conscious than he had been. Warning Joe to hold tight, I slid the needle into his neck, whereupon the colt flung his head sideways and swiped me into the ditch. I scrambled up, put my hand down to steady myself, and

19

promptly stung myself on a nettle. I just hoped that it would not have the same effect on me as it did on the horse. The head lad came forward to lend his weight on Rainstorm's head, and between them they kept him still long enough for me to get the dose into his bloodstream.

I stood back, rubbing my tingling hand, and at the same moment the horse jumped to his feet and set off with a staggering gait, dragging a totally unprepared Joe after him. They rounded the corner, to meet Mick, the blacksmith, coming the other way. "Jaysus, Joe, have you both been taking a jar then?" Without waiting for an answer, he relieved Joe of the reins and led his captive into the yard.

"My goodness, Dawson, you certainly worked a miracle there," Mr Melling beamed. "Now, while you are here, have a look at that Carol's Silver. She's got to run at Ascot and she's given herself a bit of a knock on her quarter."

I followed Gerry into the second yard where the fillies were stabled, and he led me into a corner box. This filly, I knew, was one of the leading three-year-olds in the country, and was as kind and quiet as Rainstorm was difficult. Explaining that she had been cast in her box the previous night, Gerry pulled off her rug. She had a large, soft swelling in just the same place as the one on the colt. However, whereas his had been firm, hers was soft and full of fluid.

"That's a fair sized blood blister, Gerry," I mused, feeling the swelling. "There's no chance of her running next week like that. We'll have to lance it and let out the fluid."

"We'd better ask the guv'nor first," answered the head lad. "He won't take kindly to you cutting holes in his best Ascot filly." Full of confidence from my success with the other horse, I brushed his words aside and went to get the necessary instruments.

Opening blood blisters is one of the more impressive tricks in a vet's repertoire. I only had to make a small nick about one inch long over the swelling. Brandy-coloured serum shot out in a fine fountain. I covered the wound up with antiseptic cream, and told Gerry to plait her tail and tie it to her rug in case she flicked it over the wound. Advising

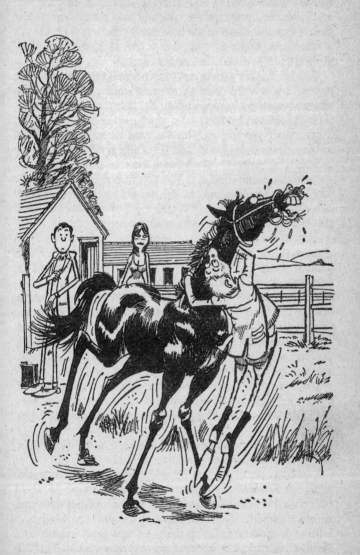

him to leave her in the box for a day, and then to walk her out for the next, trot her for two, and then canter her on the fourth, I drove round to the trainer's house.

"Come in, Dawson, and have a cup of coffee," shouted Mr Melling. "Is that colt all right?"

Feeling pleased with myself, I explained that he would be back to his normal form by evening stables. The countess had recovered her composure at the news that her pride and joy had regained his feet.

"Let me pour you some coffee, you clever man; I never doubted for one moment that he would not be all right as soon as you arrived." She gave a flashing smile, that must have turned many knees to water before mine, and leaned over to hand me my cup. As she did so, I was overpowered with the aromatic scent, which she had liberally applied, and also by the warm curve of breast revealed by her low cut dress.

Waking me from my trance, the trainer asked what I thought about the filly. "Oh, she'll be fine for Ascot, I've lanced the haematoma," I said dreamily.

"You've what?" thundered my host. "You don't mean to tell me that you have actually operated on her? Now she has no chance of running. Why in the hell can't I have some service from a decent vet, rather than you young boys. First I get one who is terrified of a horse, and then I get a lunatic who ruins a perfectly good animal."

The countess came to my aid, now that it was not one of her animals which was in trouble. "I am sure that Mr Dawson has done the best thing for her, Jack. You mustn't be so rude."

"And you can keep out of my affairs, Estella. You made a big enough scene over that black beast of yours."

The countess blushed a charming pink and, once again with tears brimming, swept out of the room.

"There. Not only do you assault my horses, but now you upset my owners," he glared at me.

Since it appeared that nothing I could say was going to assuage his fury, I swallowed my coffee and left. I set off

to little Madeline Bailey's, nursing my hurt feelings ...
There was no justice in this world. I had cured a dying
horse, operated on another in a brilliant manner, and what
were my thanks. Blast all trainers, I thought. Then a small
voice of reason in my sub-conscious offered the unwelcome
thought that maybe Rainstorm was indeed getting over the
nettle stings when I injected him. It had seemed a very rapid
recovery, even for a new wonder drug. What if the incision
in the filly's side became infected? She would definitely not
be able to run then.

Chastened by my doubts, I completed my morning's
work. Miss Bailey had not been able to wait for me, and had
left her old gardener to hold the hack. The pony with lami-
nitis at Challow had got worse since my last visit. It was not
my day after all.

Back at the surgery after lunch, I attacked Billy for not
recognising an obvious case of nettle poisoning. I was going
on about how the standard had dropped since I was at
College (Billy had qualified a full three years after me!)
and that he should have realised that the horse had a large
swelling on his side. Jim listened to all this and began to
chuckle. "Oh dear, David, did you have trouble with old
J.M.?" he laughed. "He always was a hot tempered old B
when he was the assistant to my old dad in Newmarket. All
right when everything was going well, but lost his paddy as
soon as something went wrong. I remember when we were
having a trial gallop on the Limekilns before the Cambridge-
shire. He saddled up the lead horse, and put the jockey on.
Halfway up the gallop the weight cloth slipped off from
under the saddle, and Freddy Hare had to hang onto the
mane for dear life. We all cursed J.M., and he bloody well
knew he was in the wrong, but, Christ, didn't he give hell to
the poor lad who did the horse."

"Well, as far as I am concerned, he can keep his damned
horses. I shan't go there again even if he asks me, which I
doubt." Billy joined Jim in the laughter, and I slammed
out of the surgery and into my car in a huff.

As I went to move off Jim looked out of the door. "Hey

David, that horse was drawn 6 so I put your pound on. I thought you would like to know that it finished sixth." With another convulsive laugh he went back in. I revved the car and shot off down the street. At least I would get a welcome from Jeannie. I drove to the cottage, where she lived with another girl who was secretary in one of the stables. I picked up the bag of cherries I'd brought her from the back seat. As I did so, a sticky brown mass slid through the bottom and back onto the seat. It was not my day. Even the bloody cherries had gone bad. Shame-faced, I scooped them up, and rang the door bell. Jeannie came to the door, looked at my offering, and burst out laughing. "Hey, Ann," she shouted to her companion, "come and look what my big lover has brought. I never knew times were so bad in the veterinary world."

All I could do was to grin ruefully. "Well, it's been a pretty bloody day all through, so even these had to go wrong on me."

But the two girls managed to cheer me out of my miseries, and Ann even tactfully said she wanted an early night. As I finally kissed Jeannie good night, the village clock struck one. A new day. Perhaps we would all survive; perhaps I would even go back to Melling's; perhaps he might even ask me to.

Five days later, I had heard nothing from Ilsley and hardly knew whether to be glad or sorry. Did it mean that all was well? Or had both horses got worse? Had the trainer called in some other vet? That evening I was passing the entrance to their lane as a car emerged. I saw that it was Gerry's car, so I pulled up. "What has happened to those cases?" I asked.

"Oh, the filly has done great, but the black bastard tried to eat the boss last night at evening stables. He's sent him off today to Bill Master's down in Sussex. He said that as Bill was supposed to be good with bad horses, he could ruddy well try with this one. Anyway, he would never have been ready for Ascot as he missed two bits of work that he badly needed."

24

It seemed that luck had been on my side after all.

The next week Jack Melling rang me up on Tuesday evening. He had just returned from Ascot. "You did a damned good job on Carol's Silver," he said. "She skated in today by three lengths. Sorry I was a bit short the other day, but that blasted woman annoyed me with her fussing and shouting."

"Thank you, sir," I answered with a sigh of relief. "I'm sorry to hear that you had to get rid of her horse."

"Oh, that's all right. I never did like the brute. Anyway she is sending me two others over from France next week."

Telling him that I would be along tomorrow to see a lame two-year-old, I put the phone down, and went to answer the door. "Come in, my love." I kissed Jeannie lightly on the cheek. "I've got some cherries for you, bought fresh today."

# MARRIAGE – EQUINE STYLE

STALLIONS are strange creatures. They are the chosen few of the horse world; selected by their pedigrees or from their past successes to spend their lives in comfort and considerable luxury. When I first became involved with horses, they were treated as arrogant, dangerous animals, secluded from the outside world by high fences, which were penetrated solely by their attendants and, for a few months in the year, by the mares. It was small wonder that they became suspicious of, and belligerent towards, any human who was foolish enough to approach their domain. As a student, I had been ushered into their presence on odd occasions accompanied by much caution and waving of ropes, brooms and other items of self-defence. The idea of giving a simple hypodermic injection was enough to keep strong-minded vets awake at night trembling at the thought of their probable reception.

Fortunately, by the time that I was called on to deal with these select animals, things had changed. The folly of perpetual isolation had been realised. Stallions were allowed to see their neighbours and to view the general comings and goings on the stud farms. The fences became posts and rails, through which they could watch the play of their offspring and get used to humans passing their compounds. The result was that they became more like docile, spoiled patriarchs than despotic rulers. Treatment was no longer a nightmare, although they still demanded the respect and courtesy to which their station in life entitled them. Due to their value they were rarely allowed to roam the paddocks together, and their meetings with the mares were carefully controlled affairs.

There was a particular ritual attached to work on a stud, which had no counterpart in the humdrum life of the racing

26

or hunting stables. The mares and foals were monitored hourly lest they fall prey to some accident or disease, and the staff worked literally round the clock during the breeding season. I have never known a more devoted, selfless group than the men who work to produce the future generations of the racehorse. When I began, the Captain had been in sole charge of the stud side of the practice. The rest of us had been persuaded to regard this work as something sacrosanct. Every day during the season Jim would carefully boil the various tubes and syringes which were used in the mare examinations. These were wrapped in special towels and deposited in two white enamel buckets. Along with them went two brown Hock bottles, one labelled "C" and the other with 'S". Their contents were a secret known only to Jim and the Captain for many years. Jim once caught me in the act of removing one of the corks to sniff the ingredients. Had I been found pillaging the Jewel Room in the Tower, I would not have been more roundly abused.

I had been working in the practice for several years when I was summoned to our conspiratorial dispenser. "David, old lad," he whispered, "the Captain has just phoned to say that he is ill. He wants you to go up to the Warbury Stud to see a mare and deal with her after she has been to the stallion."

"But for God's sake, Jim," I said horrified. "I don't know anything about that side of things. What on earth does he do and what are these tools for?"

"Don't worry old man," croaked Jim. "Young Johnny Fairtree, the stud groom there, is a good chap and he'll put you right. I'll put the buckets into your car; the instruments are ready and the bottles are filled." I saw my chance at long last.

"What exactly is in those bottles?"

Jim laughed, "Well, old son, the one marked with a 'C' is Carbolic solution and the other is Salt solution. I haven't any idea what the Captain does with them, but they always come back empty."

Disappointed by the discovery that our mystery had such

27

a mundane explanation, I set off to Warbury. Quite what I was going to do, I had no idea. I had seen mares being examined, but all one could appreciate as an onlooker was the vet standing in a most dangerous position behind the animal with his right arm, clad in a long rubber glove, embedded up to the arm pit in her nether regions. A series of grunts and curses were intermingled with mutterings about follicles and eggs and ovaries and tubes. Then a light would be lit in the depths of a glass tube accompanied by further comments such as "open" or "dirty", "inflamed" or "dry". No indication was given to the spectator as to the precise location or cause of these comments. Finally the operator would stand back and give his opinion of the timing of the prospective ceremony. All these valuable comments would be jotted down by the stud groom in a notebook, and then transferred to a large sheet in the harness room which looked more like a cricket score card with all its lines, squares and different coloured symbols.

This was my first venture into the glamorous world of stud farms with their inmates worth hundreds of thousands of pounds. I was apprehensive, but very excited. The weather, too, did much to etch that morning on my memory for ever.

It was the first of March. Snow had fallen in the night and lay thinly on the thatched roofs of the cottages as I drove through Upper Lambourn. Only twenty days before the Vernal Equinox, or the First Day of Spring, the sun was shining. The downland countryside was mottled with snow; in one large field lambs gambolled and sucked, wagging their little tails; and once again I thanked God for allowing me to follow this wonderful vocation in such beautiful surroundings.

Then I shivered involuntarily, not from cold – the MG heater was more than adequate – but because I was entering the spookiest mile that I know. On the right, close to the road, rose the steep, scrubby scarp of Ashdown, on the top of which, far from prying eyes, old Atty Persse would try his speedy two-year-olds. On the left, standing up from the snow, glistening with the appearance of black glass, were the tall rooky trees that surround and partially conceal Ashdown House, the strange incongruous home of the Earls of Craven.

On both sides the ground was littered with huge, grotesque boulders, formed from some form of lava deposit. The sun was obscured as the road wound through the little pass. I shivered again and thought of ambushes.

Some time later that fine escaper, politician and archaeologist, Airey Neave, explained to me, "Of course you feel it. You'd be very insensitive if you didn't. Over the years more blood has been spilled and more people cruelly killed in savage battles over that small area than almost anywhere else in the country."

Once again I experienced that feeling of relief and joy as I drove out of this "Valley of Death", over the brow of the hill and saw the lovely, welcoming, sun-drenched Vale of the White Horse stretching away in front of me. Down in the vale I branched off and was soon driving up the narrow lane to Warbury between trim, beautifully clipped hedges and smart, sound post and rail fences, which border superbly farmed enclosures and fields of rich, lush pasture, kept sweet by two hundred head of cattle. This is limestone land, ideal for breeding and rearing strong-boned young stock. Here in its three hundred acres the famous Warbury Stud was constructed at the turn of the century, since when it has turned out a steady stream of winners.

I passed solid stud buildings and sheltered paddocks, where, despite the snow, mares, early foals and yearlings grazed contentedly. Even as a young, inexperienced vet, I realised that this was equine Paradise.

As I pulled up outside the range of foaling boxes, I was met by a tall man with grey hair, a lined face, and a marked limp. He wore a green tweed gamekeeper's suit, covered by a smart brown smock. "You must be Mr Dawson," he smiled. "Old Pokey rang to say you were coming in Captain Bembridge's place. I hope he's not too bad; his poor old chest's been playing him up for years."

I shook his hand and assured him that my employer would

be back in a couple of days. "By the way," I asked, "who is old Pokey, do you mean Jim Enoch?"

"Of course I do," he laughed. "He was given the name when I was in stables and he was the head man. Miserable devil he was in those days, always poking his nose into anything that we apprentices didn't want him to know about."

I was surprised that this large man could ever have been small enough to have been a racing apprentice, but he told me that he started there when he was only twelve, and that he had not begun to grow until he was nearly eighteen. He had ridden several winners, and, when he had become too heavy, had been found a job on a stud by one of the stable patrons.

While this conversation had been going on, I had put on my long green apron and had brought out soap and a roll of cotton wool. "Young" Johnny Fairtree had meanwhile sent one of the stud hands on ahead with the precious buckets. I only hoped that he knew more about their purpose than I did. As he led me to one of the boxes he told me what the Captain had found in the mare two days earlier. He had said that she should be just right for the stallion today. The stud hand, a cheery Irishman, had set the buckets up outside the box and was busy laying out the tools and the two famous bottles. He filled the buckets with water and disinfectant and held out the glove for me to put on. I slid my hand into the chalk-filled sleeve and advanced on the mare, who had been backed into the doorway of the stable. As I approached, she swished her tail and picked up a hind leg warningly. I hid myself behind the door and craned round to reach her rear end.

'Sure it's a great long arm, you're thinking you've got," grinned the lad. "Don't bother. She's a quiet old stick now, and she's been examined more times than Father Ryan's said benedictions."

I edged closer and managed to steer my hand deep into the depths of her abdominal cavity. Cautiously I groped around for some familiar landmark. Working down from the bony roof under which I could feel her arteries pounding

30

away, I came on a round hard object about the size of a small apple. "Nothing on the left side, is there Mr Dawson?" said the stud groom. Only too anxious to agree, I confirmed his suspicion. If he said there was nothing, that was why I had felt nothing. At least he had given me a hint as to where I was in the great unknown. I wandered my hand over towards her right hip and continued my search. My fingers bobbed against another apple. Advancing my hand cautiously, all the time with one eye cocked on the mare's hind legs, I felt a large soft swelling at the front end of the apple. "I expect she has a good three centimeter follicle there by now," my guide volunteered.

"Oh quite three centimetres if not more," I answered, trying to sound confident.

"Good. We'll take her round to the horse now, if you'll follow."

The parade formed up with the mare in the van, Young Johnny and I following, and the Irishman bringing up the rear with my buckets and bottles. The door had been firmly shut on the protesting foal, whose mother seemed unconcerned by the sudden removal from her child. In fact she seemed impatient to embark on a new voyage of matrimony in a most unlady-like manner. She pulled her way to her new husband's quarters, attracted by a series of shouts and trumpetings as he prepared to welcome his bride. She was led into a small yard adjoining his box, where the attendants hurried to dress her in her bridal garb. Hobbles, boots and straps were to be her substitute for white satin and orange blossom, lest she decide at the last minute that her valuable chosen spouse was not entirely to her liking.

When all was prepared, the stallion man was summoned and the bridegroom arrived with a roar, pounding down the aisle on his hind legs, more like a warrior going into battle than a husband about to claim his beloved. He stopped, snorted, and turned to examine the spectators in the style of a new batsman conning the field-placings for likely traps. Happy that he knew all our positions, he turned on his wife and firmly bit her hind leg. She not unnaturally

31

squealed at this assault and humped her back. The bold husband, chastened by this mild rebuff, spun around and made for his quarters.

"Dear Mother of God, it's going to be one of his slow days, the old git," groaned the Irishman as he put down the mare's front leg, which he had been holding up.

"Does he often take long?" I asked, thinking of the five other calls I had arranged that morning.

"Well, three hours is his record, but I don't mind betting that he'll beat that before long. Sure an owd pig that's crippled with the rheumatics and eaten with the fever would be quicker than this idle yoke."

"Come on now, Patrick," Johnny reproved. "You'll only embarrass him more, if you keep on like that."

"That bloody old has-been is past embarrassing these days. He should be pensioned off, given a white stick and put to pull the milk cart."

"Better a has-been than a 'never-was' like you, you blooming Irish tinker," growled the stallion man, taking these comments on his horse as a personal affront. "You shouted loud enough that day he came up the hill at Epsom and beat the French horse."

"I did that," agreed Patrick. "But that was fifteen years ago. Jaysus and could I not go a great gallop myself in those days, before you bastards up here dragged all the spirit out of my heart and the speed out of me feet."

While this verbal battle was under way, the stallion showed little increased enthusiasm for his wedding. But suddenly the stud groom's small terrier wormed its way under the gate and ran across the yard. Seeing him, the horse snorted, stood on his hind legs and charged onto his wife. Patrick hastily grabbed the mare's leg again. "There now," he grinned. "It's only bloody jealousy that will stir him these days. Like his blooming groom, sees another man heading for his woman and he's off like a hare to stop him."

The wedding service over, the bridegroom was dragged reluctantly back to his stable.

"Right, Mr Dawson, she is all yours," shouted Johnny

Fairtree. I looked round and there stood my assistant with the long metal syringe poking out of the bottle marked "S". Taking it, I inserted it into the mare and made a show of emptying the contents into her dark depths. Grateful for once that the operator's movements were hidden from the audience, I pronounced that all was well and withdrew the tube. As I stepped back, it was taken from my hand by Patrick, who plunged it into bottle "C" and gurdled it about in the fluid. Reverently wiping the shaft with one of the towels, he replaced it with the other implements. I stripped off the glove and this in turn was taken and dried and chalked by my Irish majordomo. What a blessing that the Captain had his staff well trained. They at least knew the drill, and I was relieved to hear the stud groom say that he thought it had all gone off well. As I got into my car, he leaned down and said he would be glad to see me back again one day, and would I give his regards to Old Pokey.

I returned to the surgery later that afternoon and took out the hallowed buckets. "Here you are Pokey." I looked at Jim. "Fill them up for the morning. I may need them again."

"You cheeky young wretch, I'll give you Pokey! That's that Fairtree been leading you on. I'll bet he didn't let on what he was called. Fall-a-day Fairtree, we called him. Never saw a boy more often get dropped than him."

I saw the Captain the next day when he returned. "How did you get on at Warbury? Did you get that mare inseminated all right?" I explained that everything had gone according to plan, but thought it wiser not to let on that I had no idea what I was supposed to be doing with the long syringe. It seemed to have satisfied the stud staff, and, to my surprise, the mare had a large chestnut filly eleven months afterwards. So she must have been happy with my efforts. Still, despite numerous cross-questions, I never divulged the secrets of the two bottles to Billy for at least a couple of years. When the Captain retired, I am afraid his bottles and the buckets retired with him. The age of mystique and black magic was passing. My generation heralded the arrival of science and hormones and injections.

I am not too sure whether the mares actually realised the difference, as many as before managing to have their children despite our efforts. However we at least felt that we were moving with the times.

Some years later I was to have similar frustrating dealings with a stallion called The Dreamer. If ever a horse lived up to his name, it was this one. He lived on a stud which was picturesquely situated on the side of a hill. Below the main yards, the fields ran down to the bank of that famous trout river, the Kennett. Beyond the river and parallel to it, the main railway line extended for a distance of some five miles. On sunny days The Dreamer would be brought out to visit his mares, and would take full value of the delightful situation. He would stand and wait for the arrival of a train, which he could first see on his left. He would follow its slow puffing progress along the valley, over the river by the old iron bridge, and then away to the far right where it became hidden by the slope of the Downs. No matter what I or his attendant attempted, it was impossible to divert his attention from the moving iron snake, belching smoke from its mouth and blowing its trumpet at the two intervening stations en route. Once out of view he would return his mind to the problems in hand. The strange fact was that when British Rail decided to dispense with their delightful steam trains and to rely instead upon those impersonal diesels, The Dreamer totally lost all interest in train-spotting. He viewed the first of these apologies to proceed down his valley with disdain, and never again gave them so much as a passing glance.

While the stallion has to be humoured and pampered, it is not unknown for the female to be equally unpredictable. I called in on a farm near Swindon one morning to see a hunter which had injured itself when trying to escape from its field. The injury was not bad, and only needed a bit of trimming and cleaning and the application of an antiseptic lotion. As I went to the house to report on my findings, I met the farmer's wife carrying a long rein and cavesson. I asked if she was breaking in another of her good ponies, since I knew that she bred three or four useful Welsh ponies, which went on to win at the big shows.

"No," she replied, "I'm just going to use my new stallion. If you have a minute, come and have a look at him."

I followed her through the garden to the small paddock at the back of the house.

"There he is. Don't you think he's lovely?"

He was certainly a picture – a dark liver chestnut with a white star and stripe which curled away over his left nostril. He stood a full thirteen and a half hands and was full of quality. Mary Owen told me that he was a seven-year-old, which she had been trying to buy for three years. She had finally won and he had arrived the week before. Although he had covered many mares in his native land, this was to be his first effort since his arrival.

Mary caught the horse and gave him to me to hold, while she collected the mare from the orchard. "I've tried her with that old hunter gelding of my husband's and she is really well in season. I thought that she'd be the ideal mare for him to start on, as she's had ten foals and is super and quiet." She returned, leading a docile old grey with a month-old colt foal following along behind.

"You hold the stallion there a minute, David, and I'll tether Granny to the post."

I offered to bring the new horse out if she wanted to hang on to the mare, but she assured me that she always managed like this and she wanted him to get accustomed to her ways. So saying, she tied the end of the ropehalter to the base of the post which stood in the corner of the garden. Leaving the foal to its own devices, she came to relieve me of the stallion.

I stood back as she led the new acquisition off to his first assignation. When he saw Granny waiting for him, he shouted with anticipation and pulled forward eagerly, dragging Mary with him. Granny, alas, was not so taken with the arrival of her new husband as Mary had hoped. She snorted indignantly, stood up on her hind legs and struck out at her advancing admirer. Clearly the Welsh ladies had never

35

behaved in this unappreciative manner. The ardent lover stopped in his tracks and let out a roar of disapproval. This was the last straw as far as Granny was concerned. She flung herself backwards away from my desperate attempts to catch hold of her rope. With a lunge she pulled the post out of the ground and made off across the garden, dragging it with her. What I had not noticed was that the post was holding up Mary's washing line, which was fully laden with the family smalls. The sight of his intended departing at some speed, trailing assorted numbers of highly coloured vestments drove the proud little Welshman into a frenzy. He plunged out of Mary's grasp and set off in hot pursuit. Across the kitchen garden and over the lawn the motley group sped. Granny showed a surprisingly good turn of foot for one of her age, as she negotiated the rose bed and hurtled down the side of the swimming pool. This proved the point of departure for the washing line. Its sudden immersion into the pool increased its weight so the line snapped, leaving the mare with only the pole to pursue her. By dint of a short cut through the box hedge I managed to gain on the poor foal and corner it by the greenhouse. I flung my arms round its neck, and brought its flight to a halt. Granny soon realised it was massing from the chase, slowed, glanced back over her shoulder and gave a whicker of encouragement for her foal to follow. This pause was long enough for the frantic Llewellyn to catch up with his wife, whom he bowled over into the bushes at the end of the garden. Even as she scrambled indignantly to her feet he leapt to complete his appointed task. Mary arrived on the scene, grabbed the end of the long rein and secured her new purchase. Granny meanwhile was not finished, but had set off to put as great a distance as possible between herself and her ravisher. Her flight back up the garden towards me and the foal was suddenly arrested when the clothes pole wedged in the narrow gap by the greenhouse. Only then could I release the foal and capture the outraged old lady.

Later that year, I met Mary out hunting and asked her how the Welsh stallion was faring and whether she had had any more disasters with her washing. She laughed at the memory and told me that she had tried twice to cover Granny with the horse, but with no success. Each time the mare had protested violently, although she had not escaped again. She had finally taken her to a stallion near Wantage where the mating had been uneventful and apparently fruitful. Meanwhile, Llewellyn had dealt with his other wives impeccably. I replied that there was no accounting for taste and that perhaps there was a psychological barrier between English women and Welsh men. She laughed uproariously at this, and, pointing to her husband, David Owen, who was riding ahead, she said, "Well, I was born in Guildford, and that man of mine comes from Pontypool, but we have managed four children.

# AUNT CLARA

EVERY veterinary practice has its own collection of eccentric clients, and we are certainly no exception. In fact, the horse world seemed to breed its own peculiar variety of human attendants. There were on the one hand, the old-fashioned hunter dealers, who really knew horses and resolutely resisted all attempts to drag them into the twentieth century, and on the other, the afficionados from the eventing world, then rapidly growing in popularity. They were a particular trial for me, since, as soon as they bought their first horses, they appeared to don the mantle of long-qualified experts. Quite why it became a point of honour for a girl, embracing the mysteries of dressage for the first time, to become an experienced vet at once, I never have discovered. I know that, after many years as a horse vet, I still know remarkably little about the necessary controls required to make the creature go where I want it to.

Among our favourite odd-balls, Aunt Clara held a special place in our affection and nightmares. When I first arrived in Lambourn, she was already a venerable age. She belonged to that clan which had been born into better times and had slowly slid down the strata of affluence. Her father had been one of the local squires, and a considerable land-owner in the district. Since his untimely death in the Boer War, the family had disintegrated, finally leaving Clara as the sole human occupant of the family mansion. This much I had gleaned from the fading collection of family photographs which gazed down in some bewilderment at the chaos which had overtaken the house. The good lady lived on her own with a retinue of ten assorted dogs, countless cats, and a herd of nondescript ponies. Housework was not included in her daily routine, so that the carpets and furnishings had long since been abandoned to the animals.

Beneath the covering of dust and cobwebs stood valuable Welsh dressers and Jacobean tables. I always imagined that if one could put up with the fetid odour of her four-legged companions for long enough, one would unearth real treasures within the recesses of the house. In fact some years later, when Aunt Clara moved on to other worlds, an inventory was made by the local experts. Alas, nothing remained of any conceivable value. The whole house had been ravaged by generations of pets and other unbidden guests of the animal and insect kingdoms. Woodworm, dry rot, and cockroaches had succeeded where several successive bailiffs and tax inspectors had tried but failed. Clara had defied all attacks of the State's bureaucratic machine. She had finally decided on her own time of going, with no assistance from health visitors, pest officers, or other county officials. Decently and quietly she lay down in her bed to sleep and failed to greet the new day.

However all that was in the future, and, at the time of these events, she was still a considerable village character. Quite how she came to be known as Aunt Clara, nobody seemed to know. However her daily visits to the village were rarely alone. She seemed to gather a pack of school-children, rather like the Pied Piper of Hamelin, although, in her case, the bait was more likely to be bars of chocolate than a teeming of rats and a whistle. What few pence she had were spent unstintingly upon her pets and her numerous youthful acquaintances. Her visits were made on foot, regardless of weather conditions. Rain or shine, she would plod down the two miles from her "farm" high on the Downs, and determinedly plod back up again. Equally oblivious to the seasons of the year, her clothes never altered. Wearing a stout pair of button boots, a black corduroy beret, and a slightly battered moleskin coat, she would appear in the High Street with her two carrier bags. Usually these returned very much fuller than they arrived, for many of her former followers would see that their old Aunt had a rabbit, a couple of pigeons, or a picking of green vegetables to take back with her.

One of her regular points of call was our surgery. She would push open the door and, in her deep voice, shout for Enoch. He in turn would rush to put on the kettle for her.

"Such a nice young man," she told me once. "He shouldn't wear those gold-rimmed glasses. They don't improve his looks. He'd be quite handsome in some decent horn-rimmed ones."

When I repeated this to Jim, he nearly dropped the measuring flask he was holding. "Dear, oh dear," he spluttered. "Just wait till I tell my old Dutch that one."

I don't believe that that worthy woman altogether appreciated the compliment, for she said to me sometime later that Aunt Clara was going dotty and should be made to leave her house and move to a home in Newbury. Not that Alice was a jealous woman, but she guarded her husband like a mother hèn.

Apparently on one of her visits to Jim's tea-table, Aunt Clara had requested that someone should visit her to geld one or two of her pony colts. Seemingly, Billy Foster had been in the room and had immediately volunteered his services for this simple task. It transpired that Jim and Billy were not exactly on the best terms at that time after a fracas in the dispensary during which Billy had broken one of Jim's favourite clay mortars. As a result Jim had suggested that Billy set off the next morning to attend to the needs of Aunt Clara's colts.

The day after Billy's visit, I was considering which medicaments to use to cure a particularly persistent ulcer on the eye of the local master of hounds' best horse, when the door burst open and a small tornado in a moleskin pushed into the surgery.

"Where's that young Enoch?" she shouted. "I've got a large bone to pick with him."

Telling her that he was somewhere in the yard, I put her into a chair and went to find him. He was out in the old kennel, sorting out bales of cotton wool.

"Jim," I said, "it looks as though you're in trouble. Old

Clara is in the surgery, breathing fire and brimstone. She looks like having your guts for garters."

"Oh, ho," chortled Jim, bending over and clutching his stomach with laughter, "I thought we'd have a visit from her today. Did she say what she wanted?"

"All she said was something about picking bones," I answered, puzzled by his attitude. "What the hell have you been up to, you old ruffian?"

"Never you mind, David," he answered, putting down an armful of cotton wool rolls and making for the door.

I followed him into the surgery, agog to find out what was going on.

"Now, Enoch, what do you mean by sending me up a raw boy, who couldn't even change his own socks, let alone operate on my valuable animals?"

Jim made a half-hearted attempt to hide his amusement, and offered the normally sweet-natured Aunt Clara a cup of tea.

"Bother your tea!" she stormed, looking like some Eastern termagant, with her beret slipping over one eye in indignation. "You should know me better than to think that I'd put up with some young nincompoop, straight out of school."

"Didn't Mr Foster manage the job?" asked Jim with a look of complete innocence. "He hasn't said anything to me about it, and he went off yesterday with all the tools."

"Done the job?" expostulated the irate client. "He didn't even begin it. He went into the stable with my little dears and terrified them. Before I could get to the door, they were all chased out and galloping over my fields."

I could see it all. The evil Enoch had seen a way to get his own back on Billy. We all knew only too well from past experience that it was hopeless to tackle any of Clara's animals without a small army of helpers. Like the owner, they deprecated all invasions of authority, and in their eyes a vet, demanding some form of the mildest restraint, was authority. As such he was to be avoided like Bubonic plague, as fast and as violently as possible. Billy, of course, had not had the dubious pleasure of visiting this enclave before, and that old bastard had realised this and had said nothing.

"Come on now," I broke into her tirade. "I'm sure that Mr Foster didn't chase them out on purpose. He really has a way with animals. I expect they didn't give him much chance to get better acquainted."

"A way, my eye! He told me to fetch them back, and that they wanted shooting not cutting," she exploded, not in the least assuaged by my defence of my colleague.

"Well, I'm very sorry about it," I said, pouring more oil on the troubled sea. "I do know that your ponies are very sensitive. Perhaps I had better come myself, and see what I can do."

"I don't know that you'll be much better," she said dubiously. "Still you did get on with little Betsy the other week, so you might manage."

I remembered "little Betsy" with some misgiving. A spiteful old Persian cat who had seen better days, and whom I had to coax for half an hour before I could even look at her poisoned foot. Even so I agreed to come up in two days' time to see to the colts. It now appeared that there were in fact four colts in need of our attention. Somewhat mollified by my offer and a piece of Jim's special ginger cake, she set off for home to prepare for our encounter.

Later that evening Billy arrived back in the yard. "Hello, old man," said Jim, all innocence. "How did you get on with Clara yesterday?"

"Jesus, that old b——. She should be certified. She pushed me into an old shed, and as I went in, seven colts of varying ages came past me. The last one out caught me on the shin and flattened me. Then the old woman expected me to get up and chase them across the Downs for her." Billy slung his kit on the bench and intimated that someone else could deal with her. He had had enough.

I laughed. "She came in today, and I said that I'd call up there tomorrow. Won't you come and give me a hand?"

"No bloody fear, David. I bet that, if you do get near them,

42

they'll give you some nasty disease. They're as filthy a collection as I've ever laid eyes on."

"Never mind," I answered. I'll take Jim up there, seeing as he didn't offer to go with you."

"Now, David, you know that the Captain said I wasn't to go colt-cutting anymore since I had that twinge in my ticker at the McLintocks'."

"Too bad, Jim," I said, scowling at him. "It'll serve you right to die in the repayment of one of your misdeeds. I think we'd better take that Paddy Healey. I know he's on holiday from Reg Cobbs' this week, as I saw him playing darts at the Wheel last night. He's always game for a rough and tumble. I'll see him this evening, as I foolishly challenged him to a game."

At nine o'clock I assembled my team. The reluctant Jim got into the front seat, having appealed in vain to the Captain to be excused. The Captain had heard the facts, and thought it served him right, although he had warned me not to let the old boy get near the action. "Let him cope with Clara and hold the tools, David," he puffed. "But don't let the old fool join in, or you'll kill him and he's too valuable to let die for a few more years.

Paddy climbed into the narrow space that served as a seat in the rear of the MG. He was gleefully looking forward to the morning, especially since he had won three pints of Guinness off me the previous evening. "Sure it will be a change from riding those old jumpers round the road," he said in his thick Meath brogue. Like most racing lads, he disliked the boring roadwork necessary to condition the steeplechasers in the summer months, and the chance of earning a few quid from an entertaining morning was a "great gas" to him.

Paddy had been in Lambourn some fifteen years and, like Jim, seemed to know everybody in the district. Indeed, as I was to find out in later years, when he came to work for us, he was known to people much further afield. I was to be asked in France, most of Ireland and once even in the States, "Did you ever know Paddy Healey?" He was a fearless

43

horse-handler, and had been in charge of the breaking at one of the biggest flat stables.

We made our way up the bumpy road to the top of the hill above the village where Aunt Clara lived. Known as The Sheepdrove, it had been one of the main routes in bygone years, when countless flocks of sheep were annually driven for miles across the Downs to the Ilsley sheep fair. The old track led right past Clara's mansion, and what a sight it must have been for her forbears to look out of their windows and see literally thousands of sheep winding their way up onto the Ridgeway. Nowadays it was a virtually unused road, which petered out into a grass track about two hundred yards further on.

As we pulled up, the good lady came out to meet us, surrounded by her team of barking dogs. "What on earth have you brought him for?" she said, pointing to Jim. "Can't you manage on your own?"

Explaining that Paddy and Jim had come to hold the ponies, I got my equipment out of the boot.

"That's right, Miss," laughed Paddy, "Jim's going to sing a lullaby to them, and I'm going to tell them an old Irish story."

'Huh," grunted Clara, not seeing the funny side of this. "Come on then. I haven't got much time, it's egg day today. and Mr Parkin is waiting for my weekly collection."

"Just about make a good breakfast for him, I'll bet," said Paddy, eyeing the half-dozen scrawny birds, which were scratching away in the garden.

Ignoring this last remark, Clara led us over the road to the stable.

"Be God," Paddy whispered. "It would make a good safe store for a rocking horse. Anything that moves in there will knock it down."

"Don't tempt fate, Paddy," I laughed, looking up at the sagging roof with its timbers poking through gaps in the tiles. "At least let's hope she's got them all in there."

I put down my steriliser on the water butt which was tied to the doorpost with binder twine. Calling up the reluctant

Jim, who, far from singing to patients, was trying to pretend to himself that he wasn't even there, I gave him the syringe and needles and the bottle of anaesthetic. "Now, Paddy," I said, "we will catch each one in turn, and inject it, then we can catch them again and operate on them. By that time the anaesthetic will have taken and they won't feel anything. You go in first and I'll man the door to stop them coming out." Instructing Jim to keep Clara occupied, we eased the door open.

Inside there was the nearest thing to Bedlam that one can imagine in the second half of the twentieth century. The stable had not been cleaned out for many years, and the milling ponies had stirred up the dust of ages to such an extent that the inside was enveloped in a pea-soup fog. Somewhere from within came the mixed sound of struggling hooves and panting lungs. Paddy and I closed the door behind us, and stood gasping – hairy bodies brushed past us as each one sought a position further from the door than his neighbour. After a couple of minutes our eyes became more accustomed to the murk. We could see a weak shaft of light coming from a window high in the back wall, and a number of chinks struggling through the cobweb-strewn holes in the roof.

"However many are there?" spluttered Paddy. "Seems like there's fifty of the little beggars. Sure and there's one there that isn't so little." I had concluded the same thing as a large body squeezed me up into the doorway, and a hefty tail swished my face as he went by.

"Right you are, Doctor, I've got one," Paddy's muffled voice emerged from the depths as the ponies gathered momentum in their efforts to evade their would-be captor.

Groping round, I felt Paddy and followed the rope from his hand up to a pony's head. "O.K., hold tight, and I'll deal with him."

I bent down and followed the body back to the operative area. By touch I managed to inject the first colt. Taking a pair of scissors from my pocket, I clipped a lump off its tail to identify it. We managed to inject three more in this fashion. Then Paddy gave a yell, "Quick now, I've got the big devil." Again I felt along its body and under its nether regions. What I caught hold of did not feel quite right, and I was just going to investigate further when my reluctant patient gave a snort and leapt into the air. Paddy went down and I staggered back. With that, the enraged victim flung itself at the door, which parted from its hinges with a splintering sound.

I clutched Paddy, and rushed for the doorway to block the escape route. As we seized the door, a grey bullet whistled over our heads and out into the field.

"There now, Mr Dawson, you've been and upset old Martha, and let poor Viking away. Still, even Mr Grill couldn't do him when he came up during the war." Jim was convulsed with laughter.

I shouted at him to come up and prop up the door.

"Well, fancy trying to castrate an old mare! Didn't they teach you anything at college?"

I seized the instruments from him and went back into the stygian gloom. We repeated the previous procedure, and managed to create three geldings. Paddy made a grab at the last, got the rope round its head, and I caught its tail as it jumped forward. But just at that moment, I tripped. Putting out my hand to save myself, I grabbed hold of a mane belonging to one of our earlier successes. He, feeling rightly indignant at a further assault on his dignity, hurled himself at the wall.

What happened next remained a blur. There was a loud crack and then a slow tearing sound. The stable was full of flying objects, and, looking back on it, I can imagine what it feels like to be caught up in an earthquake. Jim swears that the stable disintegrated like a house of cards, and that, when the dust settled, all that could be seen was my rear pointed skywards, and Paddy's cap in a heap of tile and wattle.

When I picked myself up from the rubble, brushing brick dust from my eyes, I saw Paddy lying in the centre of the holocaust. "Jaysus, Doctor, that was a powerful dose you

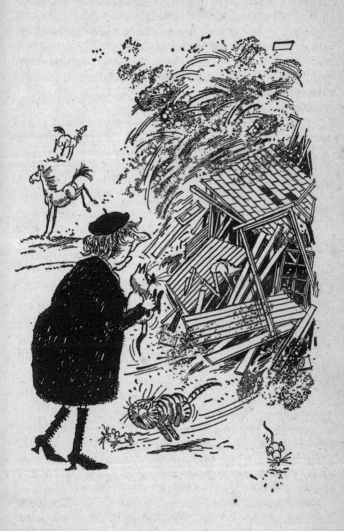

gave the last one. Had you ever better cut him before he decides to leave us?"

Where the blazes is he?" I asked.

"Well, if it's not an old pony that's under me head, the old girl has a sweaty old horse rug in here."

Pulling more rafters and more tiles away, I uncovered the final pony, trapped firmly beneath Paddy and the rubble. "Hold him there, and I'll do him before he gets up," I instructed.

"Sure, don't rush. He can't move until I do, and I can't until you lift the door frame off my legs." Remembering that my first priority was to my four-legged patient, I completed the operation in a somewhat unorthodox position, and then freed Paddy.

"Is anybody hurt?" came the slightly shaky voice of Aunt Clara. I assured her that we were all well, and released the last of our catches who, none the worse for his experience, made off into the field after his friends.

"Will you help catch Viking now?" she said, recovering her composure.

"What? And try and knock the house down next? No, I think we'll let him go for another day. Anyway, however old is he, if you say Mr Gill tried to cut him during the war?"

"Well, he must be fourteen or fifteen now. But the poor dear does get so upset by that stupid Mrs Hoskin's mares down the road. She won't do up her fences to keep him out of her meadow." With that she turned on her heel to lead us into the house for a wash.

"Thank you very much," I said hastily, "but I think we had better get back, as Paddy has to meet his wife in ten minutes."

Bidding us goodbye, the good lady looked into the car at Jim and said, "I didn't like the other boy, but this one's a bit strong, isn't he? Can you find one of your nice friends to come up and do a few repairs on the stable?"

"You don't want a repairer, Missus, you want a gang of

48

Irish navvies from bloody McAlpine's," grinned Paddy as we drove off.

When we got out of the car at the surgery, the Captain peered at us in disbelief. "Thought you went colt-cutting, not spring cleaning a brick works."

I apologised to Paddy for the disaster, but he seemed delighted and even volunteered to join us on our next surgical outing!

"As you say, Captain, we've all three earned a wash and brush-up and a few drops of refreshment. And, seeing as it's well past opening time, I know just where we can get both. I'm sure you won't be needing Mr Dawson and Jim for a while now, will you?"

Without giving him time to answer, we piled back into the MG and drove off to the Wheel.

# NO FATHER

FATHER RYAN arrived in our midst with no warning at all, like a whirlwind out of the mist one Sunday morning in September.

"Frost in May, fog in September," they say in Downland, and we had had quite a few May frosts that year.

He came hurtling down the long, steep slope of Hungerford Hill on his bicycle. He shot into the village and straight across the blind cross-roads at the Red Lion, where he escaped death by inches, thanks only to my reactions, which were quicker than usual that morning. I was returning to the surgery from an emergency colic case at Whatcombe and was driving steadily along the main Newbury road, when a black-suited figure flew right across my bows. I flung the MG to the right and braked violently. The road was dry, but the tail broke away just enough to knock him off his antiquated machine.

Some stable-lads, who had been sitting on a bench reading the racing news, went to his assistance. He got up, pushed them away and pointed to his bike. "You can put that wheel straight, if you like," he said in a North-country accent, and then turned to me. "Now, young man, what have you got to say for yourself? You want to look where you're going."

I was still shaking. "You bloody old fool. You're not safe on the road. Didn't you see that sign that says 'STOP'? It's big enough, even for you!"

Brushing off the dust, he thought for a moment, then smiled and stuck out a big hand – the hard calloused hand of a manual worker.

"You've likely got something there," he said. "My name's Ryan, Joe Ryan. I'm the Catholic priest." He saw the stethoscope on my passenger seat. "Are you a doctor?"

"No, I'm a vet. David Dawson." I shook his hand, I noticed he had said *the* Catholic priest. "But we've never had a Catholic padre in this village!"

"Well, I think you've got one now. Tell me, how many Irish would there be in the parish?"

I thought of all the boat-loads of boys brought in every year from his native country by the great old trainer, Atty Persse; of all the second and third generations, who were settled in Lambourn and district; of the Irish greetings I always seemed to receive in any of the Downland stable-yards; and I looked at those three lads, sitting by us, now engrossed in their Sunday rag which was still prohibited in Ireland. And, to my surprise, I found myself answering, "I suppose there must be nearly three hundred, Father."

"As I thought. Well, they have a Parish Priest now, whether they like it or not. There's a hell of a lot to do here and bugger all for me over at Hungerford."

I looked at him and I was quite glad that I belonged to the good old Church of England and was not a lapsing Catholic. Although Joe Ryan must have been around sixty, he had the build of a good middle-weight boxer. Medium height, broad powerful shoulders – solid. Even now I doubted if he weighed more than 160 pounds and I knew it was all muscle and sinew, no surplus. Over the "dog-collar" sat a large, noble head, which would have delighted a good portrait painter. Silver, wavy hair above a broad, furrowed forehead; prominent eyebrows surmounting wide-set grey eyes, which were seldom still and might just hold a touch of fanaticism; high cheek-bones and a strong, straight nose. The mouth was neither mean nor generous, but the jutting jaw had more strength than I had ever seen. Although obviously capable of great kindness, there was no special humour in the weather-beaten face. It was the face of a good, hard, simple man.

"Have you a Catholic colleague?" he asked.

"Yes. Brendan Dwyer is of the Faith – and quite conscientious, too."

"Then would you please send him over to me this afternoon at the Presbytery (what a word for a hovel!) in Hungerford. Meanwhile perhaps someone could direct me to the village hall. I would like to say mass."

I knew that, until now, Catholic services had been conducted in Newbury, fourteen miles away, and that the curate, a somewhat uninspiring fellow, or the Canon, a worldly lover of the best vintage port who held the speed record for mass, came to the village hall on alternate Sundays for the purpose.

The Canon had been known to announce from the pulpit in February, "No sermon today. Bloody cold. God bless you all!" and he had also declared, "I fear there will be no church in this village during my lifetime."

Strange how one man can change everything completely. One man, who had cycled all eight miles up hill and down dale from Hungerford and was obviously prepared to do the same trip regularly.

To my delight, I saw Paddy Shawnigan walking towards the chemist-off-licence, where I had no doubt he would be able to buy some booze to tide him over until opening time at the Red Lion. I thought of all that drama with his horse in the hole, the risks I took to save the poor creature; and all the money which Paddy owed us and the rest of the village. Here was a Heaven-sent opportunity to get a little of my own back while, at the same time, doing a lot of good to Shawnigan's immortal soul.

I turned to Father Ryan. "Here's the very man. He'll show you the way and you can use him for all your errands." Then, in my most dulcet tones, I called, "Good morning, Paddy. Come and be introduced."

"Delighted, Mr Dawson," said Paddy, coming over unsuspectingly. His hesitation and obvious embarrassment on seeing the clerical collar were not lost on Ryan, whose grey eyes twinkled.

"So your friend's a parson?" asked our bold Irish boy hopefully.

"No, Paddy, he's not. I want you to meet your own new Roman Catholic parish priest, Father Ryan, to show him the village hall and to help him generally. Father, this is Paddy Shawnigan, who has only two horses at the moment. And, as they're both sick with the virus, he'll have all the time in the world to help you."

If bloodshot looks could have killed ...! But the old Irish upbringing quickly reasserted itself. He shook hands. "Pleased to meet you, Father."

"Good lad," said Joe Ryan. "You'd be on your way now to the village hall to say a few prayers before mass, I'm sure. So you can take me there, serve mass for me and I'll need your help afterwards."

Paddy saw his entire Sunday morning boozing session disappearing and opened his mouth to protest. But the priest had already turned away to pick up his bicycle and was now staring intently at the three stable-lads, hiding behind their Sunday scandal sheet. They were so obviously Irish. "You three will be coming along with us, too." he ordered. "And you'll leave that disgusting rag behind in that litter-bin. Thank you for all your help, Mr Dawson – or may I call you David? I reckon we'll be seeing a lot more of each other – and thank you for not killing me. It seems I needed to be spared, for there's obviously a deal of work to be done here."

The incongruous little procession set off down the road towards the village hall and I drove happily round to the surgery where, over coffee and a good plateful of bacon and eggs, I regaled Jim Enoch with my tale of the new parish priest.

By lunch-time the village was buzzing. Brendan Dwyer returned from mass in such a high state of excitement, that he actually offered to take Jim and me off to the Malt Shovel for a pint. We accepted gratefully and listened avidly to the latest bulletin.

Brendan, knowing nothing of the new arrival, had turned up for mass at about 10-50, five minutes after the advertised time of the "off". "Those Newbury priests are so often a bit late," he said, "that I've got into the habit of being un-punctual. I'm telling you, I won't be late again!"

As he slipped into the back of the hall and joined the usual congregation of about twenty-five worshippers, he found that mass was already well under way, being said by a stranger. He was just kneeling down when the priest at the altar swung round, pointed directly at him and shouted, "You're late. You're bloody well late. It's an insult to God! See me afterwards!"

Then, at the normal time for the sermon, Father Ryan had looked round the hall and counted. "This," he declared, "is outrageous. And those of you that are here needn't look so smug. You all know who the Catholics are in the village and you're all to blame for not saving them from losing their Faith."

He turned to Jim McLintock, tall, good-looking and well turned out in a nicely cut suit. "You, sir. Are you a trainer?"

"Yes, Father."

"How many Catholic boys do you employ?"

Jim looked at Jill by his side, then back to the priest. "Seven, Father."

"And how many of them are here this morning?"

"One."

"Then you should be damned well ashamed of yourself. These boys come over from Ireland, where their old grey-haired mothers still sit in their cottages, believing in their sons' innocence. They come into this den of iniquity and they lose their Faith, because the likes of you, sir, and you, ma'am, neglect your responsibilities. You're a bloody disgrace to the community and to your religion. Catholics? Communists more like. You'll burn in hell and you make me sick!" His eyes flashed fire. A terrifying figure of vengeance.

But when Brendan, in fear and trembling, introduced himself after mass, he found a different man, firm, but smiling, the fanatical tirade forgotten.

"I shall need your help," said Ryan, "now and for some months to come. As a vet, you'll have a car and you'll know all the stables and the trainers. Your colleague, David, will tell you to come to Hungerford this afternoon. Don't bother.

54

But I do want you to see your boss and get all tomorrow off. When I arrive at your surgery, I want a complete list of all stables in the area with the names of the trainers and of all the Catholic lads, as well as the addresses of the married ones that live in the village.

"Then I want you to take me on a conducted tour of the place, show me every road and street and all the stables in and around the village. And you can help me find a likely place to build a church."

Shawnigan was still waiting. It was after mid-day and his tongue was hanging out for that Guinness.

"Paddy, you make it your duty in the next few days to see every trainer and headman and tell them that mass on Sunday is at 10-45 a.m. sharp."

"Sure an' they all know that, Father."

"Aye, and a fat lot of good it's done. You'll tell them that the parish priest expects every Catholic to attend mass and holds them personally responsible for seeing that they come. Report to me when you've seen them all." He looked at his watch and smiled. "All right, lad. You can get off to your pub now."

And so, while Paddy and the rest of us were enjoying our drinks and Sunday lunches, the lone black figure was pushing his bike up the long, steep hills and cycling back to the comfortless bare boards of the accommodation provided for him in Hungerford.

As promised, he was back again early the following morning and kept Brendan hard at work all day, showing him everything and explaining every detail of our village life. Apparently he showed interest in several sites for his proposed church, but he particularly coveted a paddock close to our surgery. It belonged to Ivor Trafford, the world's greatest trainer of steeplechasers and hurdlers, whose horses and lads were the pride of Downland. He had just married a lovely young lady of tremendous character, called Jane de Loire who, as the daughter of Lord de Loire, was a member of one of our oldest and finest Roman Catholic families. Ivor, a man of outstanding skill, immense charm and generosity, was still, like all country-born Britons, jealous of his land and loath to part with a square yard of it.

The next two Sundays kept the pints being pulled as the gossip-pot boiled. Joe Ryan was undoubtedly a star. Wherever he went, he stirred things up to such an extent, that he could never be forgotten nor ignored. During the week he ordered Brendan to borrow a long, collapsible builder's ladder and a vehicle to carry it. Dwyer and Shawnigan were instructed to be at the village hall at 10-15 a.m. on Sunday. A plan was laid.

At 10-45 about fifty people had assembled. A distinct improvement, but nowhere near the potential size of congregation. As they arrived at the hall, they had been met at the door by Father Ryan, Dwyer and Shawnigan who ticked their names off on a list. Yet another new priest was saying mass.

At precisely 10-50 Father Ryan announced, "We're off." As fast as Brendan could drive, they visited the houses of all the absent Catholics. Those who opened the door to the priest were taken roughly by the neck, shaken and ordered to take themselves and their families off to mass that very minute, or face eternal damnation for their mortal sin. Others who, having seen their visitors approaching, refused to open up, suffered even tougher treatment. Joe Ryan climbed up the ladder, through bedroom windows and literally kicked them out of bed. Mick Milligan, who already had nine children, was actually in the process of trying to create another when his bed was suddenly overturned.

That accomplished, the little party made their way to houses of every trainer and, interrupting his Sunday lunch cocktails, the parish priest reported all the absent lads and demanded that they should be at mass the following Sunday.

And some service that was! Although I could neither understand the Latin, nor make head or tail of the bells and genuflections, I went along with Brendan to watch my new friend in action.

It was some martyr's feast. Joe looked most impressive in scarlet vestments which, I subsequently learnt, he had

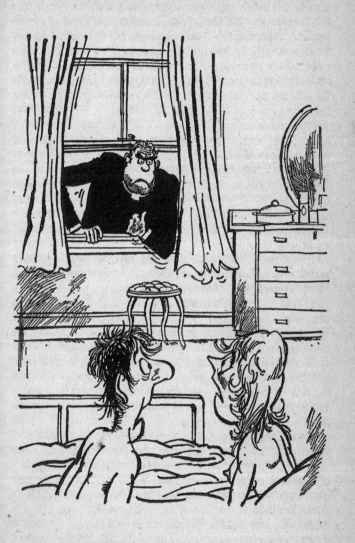

borrowed specially for the occasion! There must have been about two hundred people there, about half of whom had to stand throughout the service. I noticed that Jane Trafford, looking exceptionally young and sweet, was sitting in the front row with the McLintocks and the O'Briens.

In a long sermon, Father Ryan first spoke of the mortal sin of failing to attend mass on Sundays and Holidays, warning, in no uncertain terms, of the inevitable penalty. He ranted and roared fanatically, then abruptly, with considerable dramatic effect, he paused. After a silence he started again, now adopting a quiet voice of infinite persuasive charm. He was obviously introducing himself to his new parish and reminiscing, but his remarks seemed to be directed mainly to the front row and we at the back had to strain to hear.

"In my first parish oop in Lancashire, I was curate of a little church on the de Loire estate. Wonderful people the de Loires."

I suspected that he was putting on that North-country accent thick and strong and that the brogue did not come from the other side of the Pennines.

"I'd never met folk like these aristocrats before. But I can say this. Tha'll never find a finer, cleaner-living, more generous family in thy lifetime. 'Twas a revelation to me what the de Loires did to help our wonderful Church."

He continued to praise the de Loires (who were indeed worthy of the highest praise at all times) in uncharacteristically toadying terms, not even hinting, of course, that a member of the family was at that moment in his congregation.

Four days later we learnt that Ivor Trafford, a diehard of the Anglican Church, had given the paddock opposite our surgery to Father Ryan and the Roman Catholics.

Within a week Joe had started to dig out the trenches for the foundations. We discovered that he had found time to learn the building and electricity trades. He was going to build this church literally with his own hands. Somehow from somewhere the concrete and the bricks arrived.

Helpers (possibly under threat of hell-fire) came in their spare time and the building rose at a remarkable speed.

On fine evenings, he would work with the little remaining daylight and the glare of our entrance floodlights, putting up a fence round his property.

At that time we had a gormless cleaner in the surgery called Barney Nugent. One evening Barney stood for a long time watching Ryan at work. Finally he said, "Father, you're putting that up the wrong way round."

The priest deliberately put down his tools. "My boy," he said. "You have two choices."

"And what would they be, Father?"

"You can either bugger off now, or you can come back after work this evening and put the bloody thing up yourself!"

The harder he worked and the higher the walls of his church rose, the more he excelled himself at Mass. There was the Sunday after the death of Stalin, when Father Ryan's sermon was short and to the point. "Stalin," he said. "There 'e lies; flowers all round 'im. Lights at 'is 'ead. Lights at 'is feet.

"I WILL TELL YOU ONE THING FOR SURE. 'E'll 'ave a BLOODY GREAT FIRE oonder 'is tail by now!"

Then there was the day when, despite all his exhortations, the funds for the church building were not coming in fast enough. By this time Father Ryan had learnt all about the life of the village. From the makeshift pulpit he thundered, "For lack of money, I will have to stop building your church tomorrow. I can buy no more bricks or mortar.

"BUT I see that Vantage won last week at 20 to 1. AND I hear that those close to the horse helped themselves to no mean tune. I have seen none of that money."

He paused. There was a shuffling at the back of the church as Len Stevens, travelling headman to the stable in question, made his way out embarrassedly. Father Ryan appeared not to notice anything untoward and continued with a surprisingly lengthy theological sermon. Before the offertory,

59

Len had quietly slipped back into the church and we learnt later that the envelope he put into the plate contained £200 of those Vantage winnings.

The church walls grew.

# THE HOOVER

WE were all truly amazed. I don't think any of us had actually believed that Father Ryan could build a real brick church, roofed, fully lined, floored and electrified, with all the necessary adjoining rooms, vestry, side chapel and so on. By the time that the pews were in place, it seated three hundred. There was even central heating.

We had become accustomed to the sight of the priest in his stained, faded blue overalls and French beret since the day he had arrived at the McLintocks and their daily help, Mrs Clegg, had told Jill, "There's a dirty old man at the door wanting to see you, Ma'am. I don't think you ought to see him, look!"

He came to dinner with them one evening in late August, when they were having a special treat of beautiful under-done grouse, which Jim had brought back from York – a present from a grateful owner. The rare delicacy was wasted on Joe Ryan.

"Foony little sort of bird. Never 'ad one before. Barely a mouthful, is it? Pity you couldn't get it properly cooked!"

People held horse-shows, fêtes and various other money-making activities, but, in any case, there was obviously an adequate supply of money, because by the time the new church was finished, it was paid for. This is important, because apparently it cannot be consecrated until it is fully paid up. If your church is still in the red, then it appears that He (and who shall blame Him?) is not prepared to guarantee your overdraft. At Newbury, they had to wait for years before that Mosque thing, with its glamorous interior, was out of debt and could be consecrated.

Before the bishop could be summoned from Portsmouth, there was the drama of the altar. Brendan came back from

61

Mass in a high old state. "God, you should have heard Father Joe this morning!" he said. "He was in real winning form."

Apparently a new altar suitable for the church would cost £500 and he had no idea where he could find such a sum. But he had paid a courtesy visit to a well-endowed convent in the neighbourhood. In his broadest North-country, Joe Ryan shouted to his congregation, "I hate nuns. I tell you, I 'ate 'em. Yesterday I went oop t'convent, where they have a nice chapel with a luvly altar. When I went in to the house to meet the mother superior, she told me to put my hat down on a chest in the hall. I couldn't believe my eyes. That chest for puttin' 'ats on was another altar just like the other! An actual spare altar! Do you think that ruddy superior would part with it for the sake of God and our church? Not bloody likely! I loathe nuns and I told 'er so!"

Apparently this tirade was successful because, as if by magic, the money arrived (the generous local donor preferred to remain anonymous), the new altar was purchased and the bishop, the late Archbishop John Henry King, arrived for the ceremonial consecration.

In his address the dear old man said, "Father Ryan has built other churches and I could move him on to build another. But I think that he suits this parish. I know he's not everyone's cup of tea. He gets some people's backs up. He calls a spade a spade, never stops working and has no respect for people who get in his way, which is the way of God. In fact he's a bloomin' hoover! I've decided to leave him with you."

Joe immediately set to work again, this time building a solid two-storey presbytery alongside his church. For some time now he had been living in lodgings in the village. He still bicycled.

But there had been a time during the early days when he had a car. One Sunday, he stood up in the pulpit and announced, "I would like to thank all the stable-lads, who clubbed together to buy me a motor car to save me from cycling everywhere. It is a splendid little car and it was a wonderful generous gift to the glory of God when it arrived on Thursday."

There was a long pause before he continued, "And now let us pray to the Good Lord, our God, that the money will be forthcoming to pay for the repairs to my car after the accident which occurred yesterday, when a telegraph pole got in my way."

Father Joe was the worst driver that even Downland had ever known. That's saying something. I am old enough to have heard people say that they used to ask which road a very famous classic trainer was taking to Newbury, so that they could take the other. And in my time we used to ask the same question about eighteen-year-old Lester Piggott. Was he using the top or bottom road? We had to avoid that dashing young man.

But Joe Ryan was different. Unlike Lester, he could not handle a car – his mind was on other things. When the little Ford Saloon had suffered its sixth crash, the lads clubbed together again – to buy their parish priest another bicycle!

I suppose that we could hardly have expected a General Election to have escaped his attention, even though priests are not supposed to take sides in politics.

On the Sunday before polling day, Father Ryan, speaking from the pulpit in his toughest Northern working-class accent, told his flock, "I've been to interview the candidates on your behalf. I asked them questions about Catholic schools. As you all know, its vital that we should have enough schools in this country where all Catholic children can be educated in their Faith. None of your communist non-religious 'comprehensives'.

"Now I may not, under any circumstances, tell you how to vote. I asked these two men the questions. One of them knew nothing and wanted to know nothing about Catholic schools. The other was well aware of the problem, asked me more about it, made notes and promised to do his best for our children.

"I 'ave no intention of telling you which side to vote for. As a priest, I am not allowed to and would not presume to do so. BUT I'LL TELL YOU ALL THIS. IF YOU VOTE FOR 'IM WITH THE RED TIE, YOU'LL BE COMMITTING A MORTAL SIN AND YOU'LL SURELY ROAST IN HELL!"

Then there was the Christmas midnight mass when, flanked by the local police sergeant to see fair play, Father Joe waited on the steps of his church to greet his parishioners. When anyone, like Mick Milligan, arrived very much the worse for wear in an advanced state of intoxication, he would be told to get out and then, if he hesitated or refused, he would be knocked cold by the priest's pile-driving right to the jaw. "You're a bloody disgoosting insult to the Good Lord." Wham!

One of Father Ryan's staunchest supporters was our much beloved pony club president, Penelope Prettyman, wife of the famous portrait-painter, and as absent-minded as her delightful husband, who was shortly to be knighted.

The stories about this splendid elderly couple were endless. Typical was the day when Penelope, on a shopping expedition, had left the car parked in the square, whither James, returning by train from a short visit to London, wandered in search of a taxi to take him home. Seeing his own car, he jumped in, drove the two miles back to his house, put the vehicle in the garage and was soon in his studio, deeply engrossed in work.

He was interrupted after a while by Penelope, who apologised for intruding, but said, "James, the car's been stolen. I had to come back in a taxi."

"Dear me!" said James. "What a nuisance. I'm afraid you'll have to tell the police, my dear."

"I've done that."

"Good girl. But I don't suppose you told them to get in touch with our insurance people, did you? That's most important. Will you please make sure and do that right away?"

He turned back to his canvas and smiled. "You didn't know I could paint corgis as well as people, did you?"

Penelope duly explained their insurance details to the

police, who alerted the force far and wide about the theft of the great man's car.

Three days later P.C. Bennett arrived to report regretfully that all police investigations and inquiries had so far drawn blank. Before walking up to the front door, he propped his bicycle against the wall of the garage, inside which he saw a familiar car. He consulted his note-book and checked the registration number. Yes, sure enough, this was the stolen vehicle alright.

When Penelope answered the doorbell, he informed her, "Your car's in your own garage now, ma'am."

"Thank you, constable. How very kind of you. Would you please tell the insurance people that it's been found?"

She hurried to the studio. "James," she said, "the car's back again."

He put down his brushes. "That is good news. Our police are still very good, aren't they? We won't have to use taxis now."

Penelope asked vaguely, "By the way, how did you get back from the station the other day?"

James scratched his head. "I can't remember," he said. "I must have walked or taken a taxi."

"Yes," she said. "I suppose you must."

Penelope was a very fair horsewoman and an enthusiastic follower of our local foxhounds. Before long she had convinced Father Ryan, who had never even sat on a horse, that if you hadn't hunted, you hadn't lived. Furthermore, as the lives of nearly all his flock depended upon the horse, it was their shepherd's bounden duty to participate in order to gain first hand knowledge of their many problems. He could not be a jockey or a stable-lad, but he could go hunting.

Apparently she gave her protegé a couple of vague riding lessons before he was due to make his debut in the hunting-field, to which I was an eye-witness. When the great day came, I was lucky enough to be having another treat on my favourite horse, Bulrush, that splendid old chaser, who had fetched only thirty-five guineas as a sickly foal.

65

The meet was in the same village square, where I had first met and nearly killed Father Ryan. He now appeared distinctly uncomfortable as he got out of the car, towing the trailer containing his intended mount. He was wearing a rather battered bowler-hat, fastened by one of those old-fashioned hat-guards to the back of his usual black coat, his clerical collar and an outsize pair of baggy ladies' jodhpurs, which must have belonged to a large, deceased member of the Prettyman family.

The horse selected for Father Ryan was revealed when Penelope let down the ramp of the trailer and led out a raw-boned chestnut of uncertain age with three white socks, a pronounced jumping bump and a wall eye. "Booger's blind," said the priest. I hastily assured him that this was not in fact the case and helped Penelope to load him on to Hannibal, who stood quietly surveying the scene as more and more horses and riders turned up. The arrival of hounds, however, was too much for the chestnut, who gave a little squeal and a kick, depositing Father Joe just where he had landed when he was knocked off his bike on his first visit.

Slightly bruised, but otherwise none the worse, he picked himself up, dusted himself off, accepted and downed a large glass of port from the landlord of the Red Lion and allowed himself to be lifted back into the saddle.

My old friend, Chris Walker, the West Ilsley jumping trainer, and I assured Penelope that we would do our best to look after her protegé and we stayed close to him as hounds moved off to draw the first covert.

There had been a slight frost the previous night, and, although a fine morning in early March, it was not too bright. There was only a light breeze and we looked forward to a perfect scenting day. The bitch pack obviously thought so, too, and were mad keen to get on with that first draw. We all moved into a large field to watch hounds working. As soon as Hannibal left the road and felt the grass under his feet, he jumped and kicked with glee, sending his clerical luggage in a parabola through the air. No sooner had Chris and I reunited Father Joe with his mount than that hesitant feathering in the covert became full-blooded, deep-throated music as the pack hit off the line of one of those travelling dog-foxes found in the spring, which run straight and true. We were off with a vengeance.

By now our priest had evolved a method of holding on somehow in a sort of sideways position. As Hannibal galloped resolutely over large Downland enclosures and through gaps and open gates, all went well for a while. Then, as we galloped upsides with him, we found ourselves faced with a bullfinch fence which had to be jumped – at least that was Hannibal's idea and his rider had no way of correcting it.

"What'll I do here?" shouted Father Ryan.

"Hold on, close your eyes and pray, Joe," I said. "You're better equipped than most of us!"

He did just that, but it was not enough and as Hannibal landed over the obstacle, his rider ended up in a heap on the ground once again.

My word, he had guts. Although hounds were running fast in full cry, we stopped and pushed him back into the plate. After another ten minutes, however, disaster struck again. This time the only exit from a field was a five-barred gate. I shouted that we would pull up and open it for him, but Hannibal thought differently. He headed straight for the obstacle and soared over it with a prodigious leap which threw his Reverend rider higher than ever before, so that the final prang was even more painful than the others.

We stopped again, but this time Father Joe decided to call it a day. "Thanks very much, David," he said. "Every man to his own calling and this is definitely not mine. It's great sport though, and I wouldn't have missed it for anything. Don't wait for me. I'm not getting on that creature or any other horse again. But I'll open the gate for you, so that you can gallop on."

He hobbled painfully to do so. We thanked him and set off after hounds, but, as we turned round, we saw him waving and shouting goodbye, speeding us on our way –

from under the gate, which had only one hinge and had fallen on top of him!

Later that memorable day, hounds were running again and we were galloping in close pursuit up the grass verge of a road when a car, driven by one of our old farmers, drew upsides. Out of the back window leant a black figure, shouting in a familiar fanatical voice, "Yoicks! Tally Ho! Forard on! Forard on. Lew in there, David! Get crackin' lad! Tha'll never catch bloody fox at that rate!"

# THE GNAT

I WAS busily engaged in one of the more disagreeable chores of veterinary practice, stocktaking in the drug store. Jim Enoch shuffled along the shelves, counting the packets and bottles of various medicaments, while I noted these down in the stockbook. The monotony, and I'm afraid, the accuracy of my figures, were continually disrupted by a deep-throated chuckle from Jim, which would herald a series of ribald reminiscences.

"Three Winchester quarts of Spirits Ammon. Aromat., four Winchester Syr. Ferri Phosph. Co., two pounds Puly. Pot. Nit. – Ha, David, do you remember old Snouty Jones, who used to be at Saxon House?"

As usual, I had to point out that although I had been in Lambourn some ten years, I could not recall his acquaintances of the 'twenties and 'thirties.

"He was a miserable old devil," said Jim, settling himself down on a tub of Epsom Salts, while I put down my book to listen to another tale of the turf. "Used to do an old horse called Nero's Fiddle, who won the Steward's Cup and several other good sprints. He pulled like a train at home and Snouty was the only lad in the yard could hold him. The trouble with Snouty was that he was the meanest man on earth. He could drink beer like a fish, but drawing money out of his pocket was like asking him to cut off his right hand.

"Well, one day the owner, young Lordy Sissingburgh, was coming down to see his horse work, and the Guv'nor had arranged for Nero and two others to gallop second lot. Two of Snouty's drinking pals in the yard had taken some beer into the tack room and asked him to have a pint between lots. Snouty, of course, agreed not knowing that I had given them a packet of Pot. Nit. to put in his glass. Now even you,

David my boy, know that Nitre is great stuff for filling the bladder.

"So poor old Snouty climbed up on Nero and set up to Mann Down with the string. By the time they reached the top, he had a pressing feeling in the lower part of his belly. As they walked onto the gallop, the Guv'nor and Lordy got out of the car, and the three horses were sent off to canter down to the bottom of the hill, so as to work back. All the time Snouty was getting more and more uncomfortable and less and less able to concentrate on Nero. As they turned in at the bottom of the gallop, Snouty was wriggling painfully in the saddle. As a result, the horse put his head down and got first pull on his jockey. Gaining control, Nero went clear of his companions, and made his way flat out towards the admiring spectators. As he passed them in full cry, the trainer yelled at Snouty to pull up. Poor chap, that was the last thing he could do; he was in no position to control anything by then. Eventually the old horse slowed himself down and pulled up by the road, some two furlongs beyond the end of the gallop. Snouty slid off the horse like butter off a frying pan, and immediately made all speed to relieve the call of nature. The silly clot was in such a hurry that he hadn't noticed that the buckle on the reins, which he had looped round his arm, had come undone. Nero got his breath back and decided to move off in search of better grass.

At that moment the owner drove up in his car. "What happened? Why did you get off?"

Flustered, Snouty said something about thinking that the horse was lame and having to get off and see if his leg was all right.

"I suppose you always ride with fly buttons open," said the Lord with some sarcasm.

"You stupid beggar," shouted the trainer, coming back with the recaptured Nero, "you had better take the apprentice rides in future, you are getting past riding proper work."

The lads pulled poor Snouty's leg for days, and for the

next month the landlord of The Sawyers would only serve him half pints, telling him that his bladder was too weak for pints.

"Very interesting!" barked a voice from the doorway of the store. "If it's not too much trouble, David, I could do with your help."

"Christ, Captain, I never heard you come in," said Jim.

"I didn't imagine you did. If I ever see Snouty Jones, I'll tell him about your part in that sad episode," chortled Bembridge.

"He's dead, Captain," protested Jim.

"By God he is not. I saw him in Marlborough about a fortnight ago."

"Good, in that case I must go over and try and get another drink off him one night."

"Come on David," the Captain beckoned to me. "If we don't go now, we'll be here all afternoon at this rate . . ."

I climbed into the passenger's seat in the old Humber. As usual, I was instantly assailed by the sweet smell of his herb tobacco. The Captain settled his short, rotund frame into the driving seat, specially built up to enable him to see comfortably over the steering wheel. He gave his customary asthmatic cough, put the car into reverse and backed out into the road. Glancing over into the back seat, I saw to my amazement the old docking knife. Now this antique relic of bygone veterinary science had been gathering dust up in the loft ever since my arrival in the practice. In fact it had only escaped despatch into the dust-bin out of respect for its age, and the thought that it might one day have some value to a museum interested in instruments of torture.

"What on earth are you doing with that monstrosity?" I asked my employer.

"Thought it would be a good thing for you youngsters to see how we used to work," choked the driver. "Actually we're going to dock the tail off a filly at Jim Odgers'. She's injured her tail and the only hope is to remove it, but I shall need some help."

71

Odgers' stable was only a couple of miles from the surgery, and we were soon driving into the attractive ivy-clad yard. It was the old coach and hunter stables attached to one of those vast piles of a residence, which the unfortunate owner can neither modernise nor afford to live in. The house was open to the public, although the long dark corridors, with the constant smell of damp, had always discouraged my own attempts at a cultural visit, Mr Odgers had moved into the converted coach house, whence he ran an efficient training business in a small way. He had some twenty horses, mostly two and three year olds, which he managed to place cleverly in minor races. He usually managed to bring off a couple of stable coups a year, thus gaining the bookmakers' respect and the assistance of the top jockeys when he required them.

This particular filly was a two-year-old called The Gnat. As we pulled up, the Captain told me she got her name from her unerring ability as a yearling to kick with great force and accuracy at anything which annoyed her. On being asked how the breaking process was progressing, the trainer was told that she was lethal. "Kick a gnat's eye out at twenty paces." Not a very encouraging prospect for the person who was proposing to remove her tail, an operation which would doubtless annoy her more than somewhat.

We placed all our equipment outside the box door, and Bembridge suggested that I might like to have a good look at the troubled area. Nothing could be further from my mind, but I felt that I should show a reasonable professional interest in the case. I saw a good-bodied bay with a powerful backside and a dubious head – curly ears and a bump on her white forehead set between two small, naughty eyes. I told the lad to back her into the doorway and gingerly put a hand out to catch her tail. She gave a shrill squeal, jumped forward and let out with both barrels. Not a good start. Telling a second boy to hold up her front foot, I again put out a tentative hand. This time I managed to extend the tail slowly until I could see the under-surface. There was a deep cut across the tail root, about three inches below its union with

72

the body. Carefully probing up the wounded part, I found that it extended right round the tail. As I peered closer, I could see what looked like a piece of string in the depths of the cut. I caught hold of a strand which was sticking up, and again a pair of heels whistled past my ear. All this time my colleague was leaning up against the car, waiting with evident anticipation to see me lifted across the yard. "I think a twitch will be some small help," he said. "Then we should be able to get in some local anaesthetic." A twitch was summoned and applied with some difficulty to the Gnat's nose. She seemed to be less annoyed about indignities at the front end than those at the back. The Captain handed me a spirit swab and a syringe, loaded with local anaesthetic. "Give her an epidural, David, and then we can begin the job."

I realised that the term "we" was "collective singular". Obviously this was a case of Master and Man when the Man was expendable. As I took the hypodermic needle, a slight doubt crept into my mind. I had only once given an epidural, and that was to quiet an old mare, who was lying on the ground trying to rid herself of an over-large foal. To achieve success, one had to direct the needle some two inches into the muscles above the tail and then into a singularly small gap in the spine so as to infuse the anaesthetic into the spinal canal. Warning the lads to hold tight and pray, I plunged the needle in what I hoped was the right direction. The Gnat, taking ever more violent exception than before, leaped forward and pinned the lads against the manger. Somehow they regained control and shoved her back within my reach. I attached the syringe and pressed the plunger. Nothing doing. The pressure was too great and the end of the needle was not in the canal. I withdrew it slightly and tried a bit further forward. By this time my hand was shaking like a man suffering from epilepsy. Whether by luck or by the nervous twitching of my fingers, I suddenly felt the needle slide effortlessly down about quarter of an inch. Putting on the syringe, I pressed the plunger a second time. To my infinite relief the fluid ran through the needle and into the canal. "O.K. you can relax," I told the lads. They eased the twitch and once again two feet flashed, this time denting the doorpost beside me.

"Well done, David. Why, for Heaven's sake, do you look as though you'd seen a ghost?" laughed the surgeon-adviser.

"I have neither your courage nor your aptitude for keeping out of range," I replied acidly.

After a quarter of an hour, we (and this time I made sure it was we) returned to the filly.

"I'll hold up the tail, David," said the Captain. "And Heaven help you if she feels it."

It will probably need more than Heaven to help you, I thought to myself, as he caught hold of the tail. However all was well; the offending appendage hung limply at the end of The Gnat's well-filled bay body. While the Captain held it out, I applied bandages above the cut to act as a tourniquet. When these were safely on, he ordered the lower half of the box door to be closed behind the filly while her lad was busily feeding her with oats from a bowl distracting her attention from her nether regions. Then he gave the tail to me, and applied the docking machine. This worked in the manner of a miniature Guillotine, but unlike the red-capped Parisian matrons of yore I found myself looking away as the imaginary drums began to roll.

"That's it, my girl. Now get some dressing on that tail and bandage it all up. You had better put that on, as you will have to come and change it tomorrow." I had not so far given thought to the after-treatment. I saw that I had better work this out with some care. Finishing the dressing, I opened the latch on the door. This apparently reminded The Gnat that all was not well in the rear, since she gave one more squeal and lashed out behind, opening the door firmly into my ribs. So it was I who ended the operation in the most discomfort. The Gnat was unconcerned, conserving her energies for the morrow.

Meanwhile Bembridge was investigating his trophy with the same interest which a big-game hunter reviews his bag.

"Ah-ha," he said with triumph. "Now then when did you give this filly a laxative dose?"

The lad, puzzled, scratched his head and said that he supposed she had been dosed at Christmas. This was not surprising, since it is a common practice in the flat-racing world to give all the horses a large dose of physic on Christmas Eve. This in theory is good for their health, but in practice it serves as a good excuse for them to be left in their boxes on Christmas Day and Boxing Day. I suddenly saw what the Captain was leading up to.

Since the animals get a severe dose of the "trots" after this exotic Christmas present, it is the custom to plait their tails and tie them with string for reasons that must be obvious to anyone who has stood behind a cow fed on lush grass. In this case the string had been tied too tight, and had served as a tourniquet around the poor Gnat's tail, thus necessitating its untimely amputation.

We left the head lad to explain this unfortunate sequence of events to the trainer and left for home.

"Let that be an object lesson to you, David. I've seen the same thing happen with too tight a tail bandage. Anyway, she'll have no more trouble now. So long as some Home Office inspector doesn't attack Odgers on the racecourse for an offence under The Docking and Nicking of Horses Act, it shouldn't stop her winning any races."

Reflecting on his words, I felt thankful that that particular recent Act of Parliament had saved me from what appeared to be a not especially safe operation.

The next day I returned to Mr Odgers to renew my acquaintance with The Gnat. This time the trainer was there himself with his boxer dog. Now I had heard of the cliché about owners growing like their dogs, but in this case it was somewhat more than a cliché. In fact Odgers was a big man with a round, rather flattened face and as a result of his general overweight, he was inclined to puff and snuffle as he walked. The dog had a singular reputation in the district. To say he was a good watch dog was an understatement. He would have been a natural for a guard dog in a top security firm. He had bitten the postman at least four times, the saddler twice and numerous other people on different occasions. He had once caught the champion jockey by the elegantly cut seat of his jodhpurs, when he had come to ride one morning. The story went that when Odgers asked him if he would ride the animal the next weekend, the jockey replied that not only would he never ride that horse but he did not think he would ever be sound enough to ride any blinking horse again.

Jim Odgers saw me drive into the yard. "Hold it a minute, while I put Vivaldi in a stable," he shouted as I made to open the car door.

I needed no second bidding to stay put. What a name for a man-eater – Vivaldi, composer of the most gentle and tuneful music. I would have thought him better named after the more tempestuous composers, possibly Wagner at his most virulent.

When the dog had been removed, I opened the door and gathered my dressing equipment.

"Damned bad show, this," puffed Odgers. "I'm ashamed that such deuced bad stable management should happen in my yard. Still I don't think it will happen again in a hurry."

Murmuring something about accidents happening in the best regulated houses, I went over to the loose-box. The Gnat had clearly remembered my visit of the previous day, as she laid back her ears and swished what little she had left of her tail. After telling the lad to put on the twitch, I leant around the corner of the door to attack the dressings. This is a not uncommon position for any vet engaged in an examination of the hind end of a horse, but there is normally a tail to catch hold of to keep one's balance. Now I had nothing, except the distant glimpse of a very cross-looking horse. Leaning over at an angle which would capsize even the Tower of Pisa, I began to remove the bandages. They slid off relatively easily, revealing a healthy wound. I leant over further and began to apply antiseptic and a clean dressing. At that moment there was a shout from behind me, followed instantly by a deep throated growl. The next thing I knew

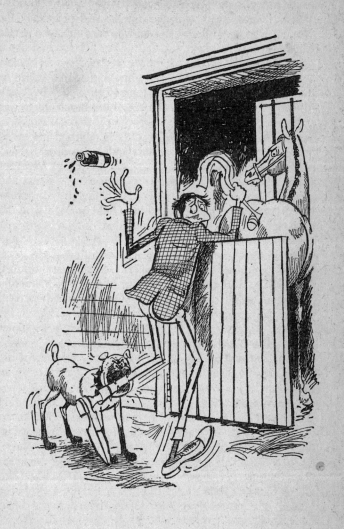

was that, added to the crick in my twisted back, there was an excruciating pain in my left calf.

"Don't move, sir," squeaked an apprentice behind me. "He'll let go, if you stay still and he sees that you're not frightened."

Not frightened indeed – with a large dog fixed on my leg, and a particularly indignant filly in front, now attached to me by a length of bandage. At least I could obey the boy's instruction. I had no hope of moving, even though flight was uppermost in my mind.

After what seemed an age, Mr Odgers returned and called off his dog. I finished the dressing with indecent haste, and limped back to the car. As it was clearly one of Vivaldi's winter seasons, I threw my things into the back seat and painfully edged into the driving seat. Through the window I told the trainer that the head-lad could manage with the dressings for the next few days, and that I would return in a week to see that all was well.

It said a lot for The Gnat's general health that she never looked back after the operation. Jim Odgers rang up in a week and said that there was no need to call since the filly had completely healed and that Vivaldi seemed to have had no side-effects from drinking my blood.

Some months later, when I had completely forgotten about this traumatic happening, I called in at a local pub on my way home. Standing at the bar counter were a couple, who were obviously intent on celebrating. I did not know them, but, as I came in, they offered to buy me a drink.

"We're celebrating our success at Newbury today," said the wife. "I had a fiver on a twenty to one winner."

"What was that?" I asked, not having had a moment that day even to look through the runners.

"A two-year-old called The Gnat. She was the most provocative sight in the paddock. What with her backside like a cook and that little stump of a tail, I couldn't resist backing her. She won easily and everybody told me that she had no chance."

Well, said, Verdi, with your female fickleness, I thought.

78

But at least she had done me one good turn. I handed my glass over the counter for a refill.

Quite unashamedly I started to tell my story of the operation, knowing that this would produce a few more "jars". It was going to be a good evening and I reckoned that The Gnat owed it to me.

# NETTLE RASH

A GLORIOUS summer day – not a cloud in the sky, and just enough wind to ruffle the long grass in the hay fields. I was leaning over the paddock rails before breakfast, dreaming of the delights of living and particularly of sailing a flying forty-foot yacht. I had spent the previous weekend sailing with some friends to France, and the motion of the grass in the breeze reminded me of the gentle swell of the Channel. The occasional sound of a bird echoed the soft whistle as a stronger puff of wind had blown through the rigging. There was much in common between yachts and horses. Both could give immense pleasure and both were, in my experience, totally unpredictable. One moment you would be in complete ecstatic control, and the next tearing helter skelter towards some unknown catastrophe. That feeling of abject terror as your horse whipped round and made off down the road with you pulling despairingly at the reins was just akin to the feeling of the wind increasing without warning to Force 7, and, having no time to put in a reef, you found yourself hurtling towards an ever-approaching shore. Still there was also the mutually satisfying feeling of relief and laughter when disaster had been miraculously averted and you tried to persuade yourself that you really had had an ace up your sleeve all the time. My thoughts strayed on until the shrill clarion of the outside phone brought me back to earth.

I went in to see what trouble had arisen to clutter up an already busy day. It was John Clearey, the tall leading flat trainer.

"David, can you come straight away? My best filly is in a bad way. Her face is swollen up like a hippopotamus, and her neck and shoulders have come up in great lumps."

"Don't worry, John, I replied. "It sounds like nettle rash.

I don't suppose it will last very long. In fact, it probably proves she is super well. Anyway, be with you in about three-quarters of an hour."

Nettle rash, so called because of its resemblance to the wheals one gets from nettle-stings, is in fact, an allergic reaction to a foreign protein. The horse is peculiarly prone to this, especially when it is eating a very rich diet and is in good health. The swellings disappear as speedily as they develop. A very shrewd old trainer once told me that, if he had entered a horse in a race and it developed nettle rash the day before, he would double his bet on it, because he knew that it was near the peak of condition. However, for all that, it is an alarming condition to see. In very bad cases the animal may experience some difficulty in breathing.

After breakfast, I answered one more call from a lady, who was worried that her cat was losing too much fur. Then I got into the car and headed for Clearey's, still musing over the strange situation which allowed me to earn money from giving advice to ladies with moulting cats, when in all probability they knew more about their pets than I did. I pulled up in the big spacious yard with its beautifully painted box doors, raked gravel surrounding a central lawn like a golfing green, geraniums, salvias, and white-washed stones. The head lad was waiting with a worried expression on his face.

"Sure, Mr Dawson, she looks as though the devil himself has blowed her face up wid a bike pump."

"O.K. Paddy," I grinned. "Let's see if the forces of righteousness will defeat him this time."

Paddy, like so many of his ilk, was an expatriate Irishman, who had never lost his native superstitions, and still was secretly convinced that the ways of horses could only be explained by the interference of the good and bad little people. A good horse was good not because of his breeding or confirmation, but only because old Seamus, who bred him, remembered to point the mare to the sun when she was covered and probably saw three lame donkeys passing by on the road that very day. Come to think of it, that may well be as good a reason as any. All the other theories of breeding pundits can be shot down with monotonous regularity. And Paddy was worth his weight in gold – a natural, who understood animals and was a wonderful feeder.

I followed him into the box, where the filly was quietly munching at her hay net.

"She doesn't look too bad now, Paddy," I said.

"Well it's a blessing that she's after eating a bit. When I told the guv'nor, she looked as though she was ready for her meeting with the Father.

There was still an oedematous swelling down either side of the face and onto her upper lip, and three raised areas down her neck, but obviously she was well on the mend.

"Now, Paddy, you go and get her a nice bran mash with a double handful of Epsom Salts in it. Once she has eaten that, I can promise you she'll be as right as rain. I should leave her in this morning, but give her a good half hour's trot at evening stables. I'll tell Mr Clearey what I think, and give him the O.K. to work her tomorrow morning if he wants."

Paddy looked from me to the filly with obvious disbelief. Still, he agreed to do as I had advised. The guv'nor, he said, was out on the gallops. If could wait ten minutes, he would be back and I could see him. Deciding that my day was full enough without further delays, I said that I would take the lane which ran up to the gallops, since I had a call to make on the Ridgeway and could take a short cut over the tracks. I turned right out of the yard and made my way up to the range of Downs which was surmounted by the Ridgeway, beyond which stretched the different training gallops. In the distance, at the bottom of the steep part of the lane, I could see a knot of people and horses. As I got nearer, I could see John Clearey's car parked by the side of the road. Behind the cars were some twenty horses, fidgeting and pawing the road, impatient to get home for their breakfast. I pulled my car in behind John's, and got out to tell him about the filly.

The lad on the leading horse saw me and shouted, "Got your gun, vet? We've got a casualty back there that ought to be put down out of kindness."

"Good God," I answered, alarm rising in me. "Not another drama already today. Which one is it?"

"Don't worry, I don't think this is one of your usual patients," he said with a laugh.

Wending my way past the fretful horses I saw a small wiry man standing beside a very decrepit old Morris. As I approached I could hear him abusing John Clearey in the most unclerical terms.

"Lorst me bleedin' livelihood, I 'ave. 'Ow the 'ell am I going to get back to me old woman and get me calves fed? Corst me a bleedin' fortune to repair me valuable car, it will, and if that ain't enough, the bleedin' pub will be shut by the time I've walked down. If the old girl don't get her nip of gin, my life won't be worth livin'."

"Now then, Bert," I shouted, instantly recognising the strident cockney tones of old Bert Watford. "You been causing trouble again?"

"No, I bleedin' ain't," he said without looking up. Following his gaze, I saw what I took to be an old feather coat on the ground by the car. Looking closer I saw to my amazement that what I had taken to be one of his wife's best Sunday garments, was in fact a pile of pheasants, all looking as though they had very recently met their deaths.

I had heard a few whispers about Bert's sideline. A true Londoner, who had evacuated from his job in Billingsgate at the start of the war, he could never resist a deal on the side. Taking instantly to the agricultural life, he and his wife had been installed in an old cottage right at the top of the Downs, some four miles from the nearest habitation. There the two of them had found their natural bent in rearing calves. They produced batches of twenty to thirty at a time, receiving them as day-olds from the milking units, and reluctantly surrendering them as weaners aged about four to five months. I had never seen anyone who could better their record at producing thriving, tame cattle with the minimum of losses. I had spent many an amusing hour with the Watfords; each visit ending with me being almost forcibly led into the house accompanied by the demand to his wife: "Get the vit a drop of gin." This was mysteriously produced from a locked room off the kitchen. Whenever I queried Ethel about this hideaway, she would grin and say that it held their retirement money. On one occasion she had emerged from the holy of holies followed by a cloud of feathers. However I had been much too busy listening to one of Bert's stories about his youth to pay much attention. Now the penny began to drop. Bert was running a little business collecting his feathered friends and passing them on to one of his old cronies in town.

"Hello, David," said John, turning round at my approach. "It's just not my lucky day. One of the two-year-olds whipped round and put his foot through Mr Watford's rear door. I have offered to pay for the damage although I think that a hole in a door is the least of the problems that old car has."

"I'm not bothered about the bleedin' car," ranted Bert. "Your blinking' 'orse 'as bruised all me birds."

"Come on, Bert," I said, starting to laugh. "Can't see that they'll be more bruised falling out of that old rattle-trap than they would have been after you had bounced them all the way to London. And anyway, if they do make five bob less apiece, it will still be a lot more than they cost you, you blithering old rogue."

Bert started and turned his watery eyes on me. "Oh, my gawd, it's you, Mr Dawson. You won't tell that bleedin' farm manager abart it, will you?"

Surprised to find that even Bert had a conscience of sufficient power to overcome his righteous indignation, I bent down and helped him reload his illicit cargo. "O.K. Bert. I won't say a dickey bird to the manager, but I might let slip a hint to the boss, if I see another load going off. You'd better stick to your calves in future." Without another word he jumped into the car, and jerked off down the road to the village, to the obvious relief of "Big John" Clearey.

"Well, that seems to have sorted that out," said the trainer. "What about Ladybird? Have you done anything for her?"

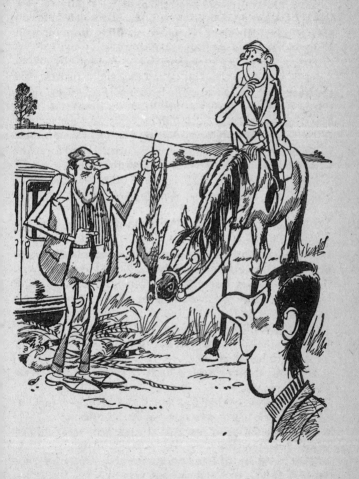

I told him what I thought and repeated my instructions to the head lad.

"You are really sure that she'll be all right, are you, David?" Assuring him I was, and that she would suffer no after effects, I left him to shepherd his string down the road home with, I hoped, no further catastrophes.

The remainder of the morning passed uneventfully, except for a large hunter treading on my toe, and a puncture on the track over the Downs. The latter really served me right, since I was about as far outside the law of trespass to be on that track as Bert had been with his birds. Still the sun was still shining. I looked forward to my lunch and the prospect of a pleasant afternoon in the surgery, where I had arranged to do a couple of minor operation with Jim Enoch.

I had just sat down with a glass of beer when the phone rang. It was John Clearey. "I'm so sorry to be a nuisance again, but that filly, Ladybird . . ."

"She's not worse is she?" I could not believe that my diagnosis had been wrong

"No, thank Heaven. But when I rang to tell the owner, he insisted on his vet coming to have a look at her. I'm sorry, but he is a good owner, who understands nothing about horses. I couldn't persuade him that it wasn't necessary."

"Don't worry about that, John," I reassured him. "What's she like now and who is the vet?"

"That's the silly part. You see, there's absolutely nothing wrong with her at all now. All the swelling has gone down and she was shouting for her lunch. His vet is Mr Parker. Do you know him?"

"I certainly know him by reputation. I have never met him myself, but he has a great name in the profession."

"Well, they'll be in the yard at four. See you then, perhaps." John rang off.

The operations at Lambourn were no problem for once. I told Jim about Bert and his pheasants.

"David, old boy, you'll never learn. It should have been worth at least a couple of brace of pheasants, let alone a bottle of his favourite gin."

I retorted with something priggish about stolen property, which hardly sounded genuine, bearing in mind the four bandages, a brand new wool rug and a headcollar which I had connived with Jim to frisk off a horse which left the yard to be trained in France the day before. We had felt that right might have been on our side, since the horse had been trained by a particular friend of ours, and had been summarily removed on the advice of a slippery bloodstock agent, who foresaw better percentages from the owner in France. Sending Jim in to make some tea, I cleared up the debris of the last operation, ready to go and meet Fred Parker.

By the time I got into our dispensary-cum-tea-room, Mr Grill had arrived with Billy. They had spent the afternoon doing teeth at Kingsclere. Billy, obviously affected by the heat and some unco-operative horses was having an altercation with Enoch about the propriety of using the zinc-covered table to castrate a kitten while Jim was pouring tea at the other end. This particular discussion had occurred many times before and, as usual, it ended in stalemate. Jim grudgingly agreed that it did not matter too much, since the Captain was out for tea and the rest of us did not seem to mind. At least it meant that we would get more than one spoonful of tea in the pot, he assured us. Alas, no sooner had he filled the teapot than the Captain's car drove into the yard. Enoch immediately coughed, spluttered and seized the pot, despite our protests. As he poured it down the sink, Bill Bembridge shouted from his car, "Send a three-year-old physic to Druids Lodge, Jim. I'm off to tea with Colonel Matson." With that he drove out, leaving us all still tea-less, and Jim speechless.

"Never mind the tea, I'm off to meet Parker at Clearey's," I said.

"Don't remember me to him," shouted Billy. "I did a locum for him two years ago. The old bastard has never forgiven me for telling a girl that there was nothing I could do for her dog, since there was nothing wrong with it. He expected me to have removed its tonsils, painted its toenails and charged her a tenner."

87

"Don't let him sell you anything," laughed Eric. "They call him the veterinary Rockefeller. He would sell sand to an Arab!"

Dismissing these remarks, I set off to meet this legendary elder of my profession. The Clearey's yard seemed full of cars. There was a big black Buick, parked alongside a flamboyant crimson Rolls. Putting my well-worn MG in the corner by John's vegetable garden, I walked through to see how the consultation was going. John and the owner, a large red-faced man in a Panama hat and tropical suit, were standing outside Ladybird's box. I was introduced. He ran a very successful line in Army surplus goods, which had brought him a house in the stockbroker belt of Berkshire, a string of horses and a demanding young wife. In addition, I suspected he had collected an outsize in duodenal ulcers, judging by his frequent self-administration of Bisodol tablets.

"Hope you don't mind," he said as he limply took my proffered hand. "I thought I would like Fred to see her, as he looks after all my horses at home and I don't like to move without consulting him."

Nodding my assent, I looked into the box, where the great man was leaning on a stick surveying his patient. About sixty, of medium height and build with pale blue eyes over a large nose and neat cavalry moustache, he wore a tweed cap, well-cut double-breasted grey suit, highly polished brogues and an old Etonian tie. He gave an impression of bland arrogance and little sense of humour.

"Open her mouth, George," he said, "and see if her tongue is normal."

George, a wizened little man in a shining dark-blue suit, obviously doubled the roles of chauffeur and general factotum. What he clearly had not mastered was how to open a horse's mouth, or at least not that of a rather fresh three-year-old. Ladybird, like any lady worth her salt, was not prepared to divulge the secrets of her age, and promptly bit poor George's hand.

"Would I ever do it for you?" murmured Paddy, not best

pleased at having his evening routine disturbed. "There now, old girl. Show the medical man your tongue," said he, deftly opening her mouth and exposing an expanse of pink tongue and yellow teeth.

Fred Parker took a step forward and from a distance of about a yard, made to smell her breath. "Oh dear! Oh dear!" he tutted. "Definite acidosis, and considerable mucous deposit over the lips."

Knowing Paddy's propensity for his lunch-time Guinness, I rather doubted if you could smell anything else at all across the box.

"Yes, Tom, a good thing you called me. I think we may yet get her right in time for Goodwood," he said, coming out of the box.

"Good afternoon, Mr Parker," I ventured, as he nearly tripped over me. "I don't think we've met. I'm David Dawson from Lambourn."

"Ah yes, I hope you don't mind my having a look. Worrying cases these can be." He looked at me absently. I was about to say that I thought she had made a complete recovery, when he turned his back and caught George by the shoulder. "Stop fussing about your hand, and go and get the number two kit from my car." George made off still clutching his bruised fingers under the opposing armpit. "Now, Mr Clearey, you must be most careful with this animal. Take her very easily for a fortnight and give her the medicine which I am going to leave you. There are three lots of powders. She is to have the blue ones in her morning feed, the white at mid-day and the pink in the evening. Continue with them for a week, and once a day you should sponge her face and neck with the pink lotion. If you are at all worried about her, give me a ring and I'll see her again. I'm sure Dawson won't mind. Always learn something from an old dog, eh, my boy?" he finished with a deprecating grimace to me. George returned with a box full of powders and lotions which looked sufficient to treat every animal in the stable. Once the medicines had been offered up, the visiting party departed, satisfied with a good job done.

Paddy turned to me as he shut the box door. "Jaysus, and wouldn't he have been a holy terror selling brushes round the houses? My old girl would have bought this year's supply off him and never known she had had a choice!"

They had all told me Fred Parker was a great business man, but I still never believed it was possible to prescribe so many drugs for a healthy animal.

When I returned to the surgery that evening, Billy asked me if I was impressed with his ex-employer. He had certainly made an impression on me, but I was not sure it was a favourable one. If that was what it took to get rich, I decided that honest poverty had its virtues. At any rate, the wretched Ladybird would not dare to get nettle rash again for a few days.

As it was, John tried to keep her quiet, but after three days she was so fresh that he had to give her some work. When I saw him three days later, I asked how she was.

"Perfect. I'm going to run her at the end of this week."

"What about her prolonged rest?"

The tall trainer's eyes twinkled and he smiled mischievously. "I rang the owner and told him that she had done so well on Mr Parker's excellent medicine, that she'd already made a complete recovery."

Some months later I was reminded of the incident. I was in Clearey's stable for another horse and went into the feed room to find Paddy. There on the shelf was a large collection of blue, white and pink powders.

"Didn't you give that filly those powders from Parker?" I asked.

"Sure, I gave her some the first night, Mr Dawson, and niver a mouthful of her food did she touch. I told the Guv'nor and he said I was to carry on with the Epsoms, but sure I wasn't to tell the owner, until maybe when she had won a decent race. But when she won at Newmarket last week I hadn't the heart to tell the poor man. So I kept them in case that medical man comes again so he needn't empty his car a second time."

# POTTED VET

NAMING your own animal has always been one of the pleasures of buying yearlings. I deplore the French habit of naming them before they go to the sales. A good horse deserves a good name. The great showmen have always known this. What judge could fail to look at a show hack called Liberty Light or a heavyweight hunter called Mighty Fine or Mighty Atom?

You can frequently work out a satisfying combination of the names of the sire and dam. So the produce of The Solicitor and Reverie might be Silence in Court and an animal by The Solicitor out of Rue Royale could well be called Judgement of Paris. Blandford, Gainsborough, Sir Ivor, Mill Reef, these are the names of the good horses. Like the first two of that quartet Grundy comes from the hound list, which I strongly recommend to those in doubt. It contains an alphabetical record of splendid, dignified names with the accent on the first syllable for calling.

But it is surprising how many bad names there are. Winagain never won and Passifyoucan was always being passed. There are, of course, exceptions to the rule, although Hard to Beat may not be pushing your luck too far. Perhaps only that great French breeder and wonderful lady, Mme Elizabeth Couturie could get away with calling a horse Right Royal. If most of us had done this, the colt would smartly have found its way to a selling hurdle at Wye.

But then Mme Couturie is one of the few remaining people with the gift, possessed by some old stud grooms, of being able to tell within the first twenty-four hours of a horse's life if it is destined to be a great horse. One morning when the Marquess of Waterford was staying with her, she came in to breakfast after her usual morning visit to the stables. "Tyrone," she said. "That colt that was foaled last night will not only be the best of this year's crop of foals; he'll be a really good horse. Do you mind if I call him Tyrone after you."

So she knew that Right Royal would be a champion worthy of his name just as surely as Dick Dawson saw a great horse in the tiny new-born colt he was to name Blandford.

Under a new rule a name, once registered, cannot be changed after the horse has run under rules in any country. This can lead to complications when horses are sold and to some embarrassment when a horse that carries the name of a famous firm or product turns out to be useless.

Bob Boucher, one of the luckiest owner-breeders in the game (Wilwyn, Fleet, Realm, etc.) recently bought back a two-year-old brother to the useful Padlocked. To Bob's horror he found that the colt which he had bred and of which he was now, once again, the owner, had been named Lovelace Watkins.

"I gather that this is some pop singer," said the famous old fruit farmer. "So I wanted to have the name changed. But Weatherbys informed me that, as the colt had run in this name, he must keep it, under the new rule. I wrote to the senior steward of the Jockey Club, but he replied that, as the name was apparently not obscene, nothing could be done about it!"

The Irish, who sometimes present horses with extraordinary names, have perpetrated some real horrors, including Boys Hurrah!, Big Bugs Bomb and Elsie's Gonebananas. By comparison the McLintocks' latest importation, a moderate liver chestnut jumper called Bog Wheel, was mild. He turned out to be rather slow due mainly to a very straight shoulder and the smallest bit scatty like many of his colour, but quite harmless and indeed he was a very kind horse. Everybody loved him and he became a great character. During the winter when he was clipped out, "Boggy", as he was soon called, was a funny sight. He steadfastly refused to allow anyone to clip his head, which consequently remained very woolly and, after my experience with Jeremiah, the cob, I didn't push myself forward or insist on the use of tranquillisers. Anyway they were quite happy with him as he was and his comic appearance merely enhanced his popularity.

Then one day Jim summoned me. "I'm worried about Boggy, David. He's such a bad do-er. If he won't eat a bit more, I'll never get any real condition on him. We've wormed him and you did his teeth soon after he came over from Ireland. He seems well enough in himself, but I think he's a worrier."

After inspecting the horse thoroughly and finding nothing wrong, I was inclined to agree. "Why not have a word with the people who had him in Ireland? After all, his form wasn't too bad over there."

The following morning I didn't like the mischievous smirk on Enoch's face.

"Now, what is it?" I asked.

"Just had Mrs McLintock on the phone," he said blandly. She'd like you to find her a goat, please, David, as quickly as possible. It's very urgent!"

"A goat? What on earth . . ." I dialled the McLintock's number. "Jill, it's David. What's all this about a goat? I'm not a farmer."

"No, but you are a vet and I know that you'd like to cure poor Boggy. He must have a goat. No wonder he's been worrying. Jim telephoned Ireland last night as you suggested and discovered that Boggy always had a goat for company wherever he went. It slept in his box with him."

"Much as I'd love to help you, I can't get goats into my MG. But, if you ring Bert Lammin near Abingdon, he may be able to help. He's got quite a few goats on the farm."

The next time I called in at the little yard, it was between lots on a sunny summer morning and all the lads were gathered round happily watching a boxing match. One of the greyhounds was sparring with a brown-and-cream coloured nanny goat. It was a pretty sight and made an amusing cabaret.

Apparently Nanny and Boggy had settled down well together and were such bosom pals that the goat had to be forcibly restrained from following her companion when he went out with the string to the Downs. I was assured that Boggy was doing much better now, eating everything he was given, licking out his manger.

"That was obviously the answer," said Jim. "It's worth remembering the next time that you have a worrier, David. Get a goat."

However the weeks went by and, although his manger was still licked clean morning and evening, Boggy refused to put on any condition. I wondered . . .

I asked Jim to take Boggy out second lot and arranged to be in the yard soon after midday when the horses were done up, watered, fed and let down for their afternoon rest. All the lads left for their dinners, the headman checked that every box door was closed and properly bolted and then left for his own cottage. I asked myself in for a drink with the trainer and his wife.

"You're very mysterious, David," said Jill. "What are you plotting?"

I just laughed. After a quarter of an hour I put down my drink and said, "Come with me very quietly."

We tip-toed back into the yard and I led the way to Boggy's box where I looked cautiously through the window and then beckoned Jim and Jill to do likewise.

"There's your answer," I said. "No wonder it's not the horse that's putting on weight."

Standing right in the manger, guzzling away and wagging her little tail was Nanny. As soon as she saw us looking, she leapt down guiltily. I don't believe that she ever really forgave me for discovering her secret. However there was no chance of parting her from her friend. Boggy created such frightful scenes whenever she was absent, that the goat even had to go to the races with him.

This secured a very happy arrangement, although a nuisance for Bill, the travelling headman. Then one day at Fontwell Boggy had a hard race, was beaten and came

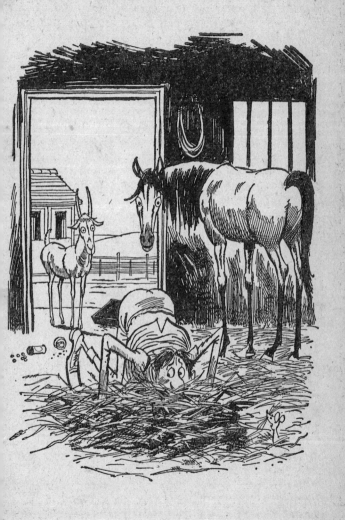

back to his box still in a state of rare excitement. Normally, when he made little diving nips at her, Nanny dodged out of the way. This time he was just too quick for her. Snap! Without really knowing what he was doing, he had bitten off her ear. I dressed her when she arrived home that night and I think that, when the antiseptic stung, she resented me more than ever.

Now Bog Wheel, with his one-eared goat, became even more of a celebrity. The inseparable pair were photographed for the picture papers and one day they were even featured on television.

However the day that I went up to give the McLintock horses their flu injections, I had other things on my mind and, even if I noticed that Nanny was not in the box with Boggy, I probably assumed absently that she was round the back of the feedbox, helping herself to illicit grub. As I went from box to box, I would put my instruments and the serum in each doorway. Suddenly when I bent down to pick up my syringe there was a roar of laughter. Before I could straighten up I was butted hard in the backside by a hurtling goat and launched painfully in an ignominious heap under the manger of a quite unperturbed Bog Wheel who, I swear, winked at his friend.

As I picked myself up shame-facedly, the McLintocks and their lads were weak with laughter.

"She lined you up and aimed you," said Jill helplessly. "It was so clever of her. I hadn't the heart to warn you!"

Jim was wiping his eyes. "She actually potted you!"

Funnily enough, although she butted more people from time to time, Nanny never had another go at me. I think she reckoned that she owed me that one and had bided her moment. Now honour was satisfied. It had a remarkable effect on Boggy, whom I had long suspected of possessing a warped sense of humour. From that moment his condition and consequently his form improved and he never looked back. Unlike me. I always do before I bend down to pick up anything nowadays!

# TEDDY

WHEN popular jump jockey, the Honourable Edward Cubitt,
bought a stable in my area and set up as a trainer, he fell
under my wing. In the early days it was more the case of my
being under his. He was a man of great self-confidence,
enormous charm for those who he liked, and total impatience. The first time I walked into his yard, he turned from
the drain which he was busy unblocking, looked me up and
down and said, "So you're the vet, are you? Never believe
what vets tell me. They're the world's greatest pessimists.
Always say that the horse shouldn't run and needs at least
seventeen injections, all of them more expensive than the
last."

Not a very encouraging start, but I immediately decided
that attack was going to be the best form of defence in this
case. "Don't you believe it," I said. "You can run them as
often as you like, so long as you can deal with the owners.
Anyway, I don't care for filling horses up with drugs. I have
always believed that nature is best, allowing that we can
give her a helping hand along the way."

So the ice was broken and Teddy, as he was universally
known on the racecourse, showed me round his new yard
with its five recently purchased occupants. I admired each in
turn, but, coming to a flashy chestnut colt in the third box, I
ventured that he was a bit short of bone and a little straight
in his fore-legs. As I got no answer to this, I felt the legs. "He
won't want hard ground," I said, looking up at my new
client.

"What did you say?" he asked. "I'm deaf, and I can only
hear what I want to."

I chuckled. I suppose he was like that good jockey, the
late Eph Smith. He was deaf in one ear and even wore a deaf
aid. But, the story went that a stable lad asked him for a

fiver after his horse which Eph had ridden had won a race. Smith said, "No good talking into that ear. Come round the other side to the two bob window, and I might be able to understand."

I was to discover that Teddy was able to make the greatest use of his deafness, which had originally started from standing too close to a German hand grenade during the last war. A Grenadier Guard, he had been one of those dashing irresponsible young officers, who were at once the despair and delight of their superiors, the driving force in the success of the British Army.

Now he was to become the despair of authority and of his owners, but nevertheless a highly successful trainer. Orthodoxy was anathema to him. He argued that trainers had for generations followed a pattern of training, and that it was time someone tried a new approach. In this he had a ready accomplice in me. I had for some years wondered why horses ran no faster than their predecessors, whereas in human athletics, records were broken annually.

My first visit ended in my persuading him to try some Sulpha powers on a four-year-old, which had all the signs of a sinus infection. He grudgingly agreed to feed these to the horse, asked me in for a glass of Scotch, and then disappeared back down the manhole from which I had disturbed him. I felt that at least working with Teddy would not be dull.

Some days later I called back at the stables to rasp the horses' teeth. The trainer met me in the yard. "Hello, David," he shouted. "Come to cause more trouble, have you?"

"Well, I can't do much harm with a tooth rasp, you know."

"You don't have to shout I can hear you all right when I need to," he grinned. "That sinus case got better, but I don't think it could have been your powders, as I steamed him with Balsam at the same time and that must have done him good."

"Never mind, so long as he is better," I replied. "Let's get these teeth done."

He led me round to his head lad. "Don't listen to Fred. He doesn't believe in doing teeth. He has never been to a dentist in his life. One look at his mouth can prove it." Fred was a short burly man with a dirty old checked cap perched on top of a mop of unruly hair. In a broad Yorkshire voice, he welcomed me and gave a lop-sided, virtually toothless, grin.

I finished the dentistry and was putting my tools back in the car, when a horse-box arrived at the yard entrance.

"Brought that filly, have you mate?" Fred called to the box driver.

"Yes and you're bloody well welcome to her. She's a right cow and no mistake," said the driver sourly. He let down the ramp and Fred went up to lead out the new arrival. As he put his hand out to untie her rope she let out a squeal and I heard the partition crack as her hind legs thumped into it. Fred did not appear to notice her disapproval. As he started to come down the ramp and put a foot on the sloping matting, the filly coiled her hind legs under her body and gave a leap into space. Fortunately, Fred had attached a long lunge rein onto her headcollar, and she pulled up in the corner of the yard at the end of the rein.

"Happen she's a bit lively," said Fred with a laugh. "Never mind, love, we'll soon have you quiet and friendly." He took in the rein and gradually approached her, talking soothingly all the time. The chestnut stood, four square, watching him advance. Suddenly her ears went back, and her mouth opened as she lunged forward to meet him. My warning shout was too late, as Fred stumbled and dropped the rein. The furious animal set off up the yard with a snort. At this moment Teddy came out of his cottage. "Ah, good, I see that the Nasrullah filly has come then. What are you all doing? Surely there's no need for you to start lungeing her already?"

By now the new arrival had taken herself up into the corner by the muck pit. Teddy grabbed a handful of carrots from the food shed as he passed and walked straight up to her. To our amazement, she stood still, watching him allowed herself to be tempted by a carrot and was finally caught.

"Put her in the end box, boss, next to the hack," said Fred, watching his employer with mixed feelings of disbelief and admiration. Teddy led her into the stable and undid the buckle of the rein. With that she reared, gave a squeal and lashed out at the wall."

"I told that builder that chip board wouldn't last very long. He said he'd guarantee it for three years, so that's one piece he'll have to put back for nothing." Looking over the door, I could see where one whole side of the boarding was split with two round holes, neatly punched by the hind hooves.

"You will have to watch her, Fred. The owner tells me she is a bit useful with her hind legs," warned Teddy.

"Aye, she's not too slow with her front either," grunted the head lad. "Have they done anything with her at all, boss?"

"Not unless they could help it, I gather. She went to Newmarket to be broken and they sent her back as unmanageable. How do you think that we came to have a well-bred two-year-old like this?" Teddy went on to explain that her owner usually had his horses trained by one of the most fashionable flat race stables. When they returned this particular one, he had phoned Teddy, with whom he had soldiered in the Army, and had suggested that he might like to try and tame her.

I heard no more about the man-eater for some weeks, except that her trainer announced that she was coming on slowly. Meanwhile Teddy had started the season well, winning four races, including both a hurdle race on Easter Saturday and a maiden flat on the Monday with the same four-year-old, presumably recovered from his sinusitis. Three of his yearling purchases had all acquitted themselves well, two winning and the third finishing a creditable second.

One afternoon I was working in a stable in the district, when the phone rang. The owner came out of the house and told me that there was an urgent call for me to go to Mr Cubitt's. I finished dressing a hunter's leg, which had been badly gashed when the horse had taken fright in a thunderstorm, and set off to cope with the emergency.

Pulling up outside the gate, I saw Teddy waiting in the feed room. "Glad you got here quickly. I am afraid we've got a nasty injury, but it should only want a few quick stitches." Teddy gave a wry grin and said that he was sorry, but it was her. The lad had been cleaning her box out, when she suddenly lashed out at him and caught her hind leg on a prong of his fork. "Never mind," he said. "It's a clean cut. The prong must have gone in alongside her tendons and come out by the side of the cannon bone. By the way, just to encourage you, she's got a name now – Spiteful Kate."

I thanked him for this extra confirmation of her sweet nature and went in to see her. She was holding up her near hind leg, clearly in some pain.

"At least she's no hind shoes on," I remarked to the lad.

"We only got the front ones on last week and that took the blacksmith an hour." He had then understandably refused to tackle the back ones since she had punched three more holes in the side of her box. I approached her gingerly, and put a hand on her quarters. She gave a squeal, and I jumped back out of the box. Not a good start. Telling the lad to push her backside up against the wall, I tried again. This time I managed to pick up her leg and could see there was a flap of skin hanging from a cut about three inches long. The sensible thing to do was to give her an anti-tetanus injection, puff on some antiseptic powder and bandage it up. However, to my complete amazement, I heard myself saying to Teddy that I would put in about four sutures which would make a better job. The trainer was delighted by this, although I got the impression that Fred and the lad were not so enthusiastic.

Inwardly cursing my foolhardiness, I went off to get a tranquilliser in the hope that it would make my patient accept, even if not actually enjoy, my ministrations. I inserted the needle in her neck. As soon as she felt the prick, she catapulted herself round the stable. The three of us became enmeshed in each other's legs and the straw in our

101

anxiety to get as near to the door as we could without actually letting her go. Grabbing hold of her again, I tried to fit the syringe on to the needle. Once again she set off in an impressive imitation of a bucking bronco.

"Give me a leg up on her doc, and I'll keep her still," the lad volunteered breathlessly. Dubiously I threw him onto her back. To my surprise, she settled.

"O.K., now take the syringe and see if you can get it onto the end of the needle from there." I handed it up to him and, to my relief, he fitted it on and pressed home the plunger. Stage one completed. I suggested we leave her for a quarter of an hour, during which time I could boil up my instruments and get everything ready.

I went into the kitchen and put the steriliser on the stove. I found Teddy in the sitting room nonchalantly having a cup of tea. Quite unconcerned, he was reading the evening paper with his pet parrot sitting on his shoulder. He glanced up as I came in, "Finished all right, have you?" He grinned.

"Christ, what an optimist," I exploded. "It's taken us this long to get a needle in her neck, let alone into her hind leg."

"Pretty Kate, pretty Kate," screeched the parrot.

"And what's more your parrot isn't much of a judge of horses if she thinks that wildcat is a pretty animal." Teddy laughed and explained that the bird was called Kate, and he had named the filly after her, as he knew she too would grow to love him.

"Now, you can come and see just how far that love has grown. You hold her and I'll stitch her," I urged.

"What did you say, David?" he smiled.

I caught him by the shoulders, and hauled him out of the chair, as I repeated my suggestion. He gave a resigned shrug, and followed me out. "Hold on a second," he shouted after me, as he ducked back into the room.

I returned to the filly, who did not look much more tranquil than previously. Filling my syringe with local anaesthetic, I advanced on her. Teddy followed me in, beckoning the lad to leave. This he did with indecent haste. I noticed that the trainer had a paper bag in his hand, from which he drew a brown sticky object, which he offered to the filly. She sniffed it and then began to chew on it.

"Get on then David. She will be no trouble now."

I leant down, picked up the injured leg, and put the syringe on the straw. I removed the needle, noticing with some surprise my apparent inability to keep my fingers steady. With a quick thrust I pushed the needle over the nerve above the cut. The filly, thank Heavens, did not rear, but only jumped forward with me hanging on to the end of her leg. Somehow I managed to get in a large dose of local and repeated the manoeuvre on the inside of the leg. Now the whole stable staff were gathered at a respectful distance around Kate's stable, waiting for the fireworks. "Good luck, sir," one of them offered. "I'll send you some roses in hospital."

After a while I tenderly touched the wounded area. I seemed to be feeling it more than the patient, so I proceeded to sew the edges of the wound together. This was easier said than done, since I found that I developed an alarming crick in my back by bending over at arm's length from the scene of the operation. Finally I got it all tidied up, put on a crepe bandage and was just about to put a length of gauze bandage over the pin, when she plunged forward without warning.

"Sorry about that," Teddy remarked, as he extricated himself from the hay net. "I've run out of toffees. Anyhow, it looks as though you've finished. I shouldn't worry about the bandage. I am sure Fred won't be in a hurry to change it." So toffee was the clue to success. Teddy admitted that he had been through all the sweets at the local shop before he could find Spiteful Kate's favourite.

I viewed the injury a week later from a safe distance. Thankfully it had healed well. She seemed none the worse for her experience, although she was so bad before, that there was not much room for her to become more difficult. She never did have any hind shoes on, and eventually won three races as a three-year-old. However, she only achieved victory after becoming pregnant to a local horse. The state

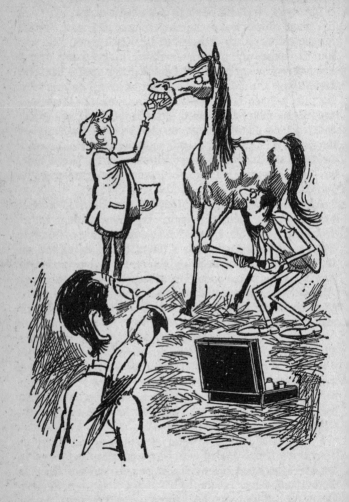

of incipient motherhood had a greatly improving effect on her mental and physical processes, as it does with the fillies of this type. And, although, to humans, it may seem wrong to race a pregnant woman, many mares, no longer worried about their nether regions, show the best form of their lives and in the early months, there is no risk to foal or mother.

I was to have little more trouble from the filly during her training period. However, some years later I happened to be on a stud, when I saw the stud groom emerge from a foaling box looking as white as a sheet. He told me that he had just caught hold of the worst mare that he had ever had any dealings with. She had arrived in foal and had defied all attempts to catch her for three weeks. Whenever anyone went into the box to feed her, she ran at them with her mouth open. At last he had caught her in the act of producing a fine colt and had managed to get a length of rope on her headcollar. Even then she had taken time out from the birth process to get up and try and kick him up into the rafters. Asking her name, he mentioned my old friend from Teddy's. I laughed and suggested a pound of toffees. Alas, it appeared that not only had the thrill of motherhood worn off, but also the lure of toffee. To add insult to injury, her new owner had sympathised with the groom for the trouble the mare had given him. He then presented him with an envelope, containing a miserable offering of ten shillings. This he suggested should be invested on one of his two-year-olds which was running at Goodwood next day. The stud groom duly invested his hard-earned present at the ungenerous odds of six to five, and the two-year-old was soundly beaten. Once again Spiteful Kate had the last laugh.

As I mentioned earlier, Teddy was keen to try any new theory which might improve his horses. A year later I went to a veterinary conference at which we were addressed by a medical expert from the world of athletics. Fired by his enthusiasm, I bought a couple of books on modern methods of training. This was the era of Gordon Pirie, when British middle-distance athletes were leading the world, following the trail blazed by Roger Bannister and Chris Chattaway.

Interval training was the current recipe for success. I could not wait to appraise Teddy of my new theories. He, as I had hoped, reacted enthusiastically. There was, however, one great drawback in transposing human methods to the equine field. All athletic training takes place on a circular track, whereas racehorse gallops are usually straight.

Teddy seized my books and decided that the problems confronting him were minuscule compared with the likely benefits from the improved training methods. By now he had forty horses under his care, and his exercising schedule was in no way orthodox. It was no surprise to find twenty horses doing a steady canter up one of the steep hills round his village. This in itself would not have been noteworthy, but, in his case, they were on the tarmac roads, usually at least three abreast and not in any obvious control. Without a circular gallop, Teddy reasoned that he should walk his horses for a furlong, canter them for the next furlong, and so on to the top of the gallop. Once there they would run round and repeat the procedure down the gallop. This could have been all very well, if he had had the gallop to himself. But he was only a tenant there, and the owner preferred to work his horses in a more orthodox manner. On the third morning there was a major confrontation. Seventeen of Teddy's horses came over the brow in a one furlong dash, to meet eleven of the landlord's cantering up the correct way. The shouts of the jockeys mingled with the abuse from the offended trainer could be heard down in the village. Teddy, not unnaturally, turned his deaf ear, and shouted to his head lad. "Mr Bancroft seems very vocal this morning. Is he congratulating me on our double yesterday?"

"No, sir," warned Fred. "I think he muttered something about hell and damnation, bloody fool amateurs, and solicitors in that order."

"Never mind," responded Teddy. "We'll send him round a goose this afternoon. I managed to shoot one yesterday, when it flew over the paddock fence. "But that belonged to Mr Bancroft, boss. You know he's got a flock of them to guard his stables."

"Never mind, at least we can save him the trouble of plucking it!"

This was the end of the interval training, but not of Teddy's disregard for normal training customs. Indeed over the years he was to disillusion me on many of my long-held beliefs. He would run horses with the most unpromising legs and joints, vowing that a race would do them good. I was continually surprised at how many times he was right. He took the same view as another good friend of mine, Monty Jones.

"Keep running them. If you give a racehorse a holiday, ten to one he'll get in some sort of trouble." He once showed me a good two-year-old with a nasty swollen front fetlock. "What should I do with him then, David?"

"Poultice it, and then apply a working blister for ten days."

"Nonsense," came the reply. "I'll run him at Epsom in a couple of days and he'll win." He did. The horse won *and* came home with his joint better than before.

We were very sad when Teddy moved to Newmarket. I missed him particularly badly. The following summer I had just pulled up in the car park at Yarmouth, when a powerful, hotted-up Ford Cortina drove in beside me. Although it was only a few months old, the engine was banging away like a steam-hammer.

The driver's face lit up when he saw me. "Hallo, David," he shouted above the din. "Killed any good horses lately?" He switched off.

"Good to see you, Teddy. That car of yours is sick enough. You've run a big end."

Teddy smiled. "That's the advantage of being deaf. I can't hear it. Splendid cars – Fords. You never need to put in any oil or water. When they go wrong as you say this one has, it always seems to happen well within the guarantee time. So I change them in for new ones!"

# A BIT OF GINGER

GINGER GRAFTON has been my great friend for so long now, that it is hard to describe him objectively. Small, lean, wiry and tough as whipcord, he had, as a cavalry officer, ridden successfully as an amateur during the golden thirties. His nickname came naturally from the colour of his hair and from his fiery temper. But this is a genuine case of bark being worse than bite. That intimidating scowl conceals an infectious, albeit reluctant smile and a twinkle in the eyes, now partly hidden behind half-glasses that sit below a pair of thick sandy brows.

At the time I joined the practice, Ginger was training a small string of horses with canny skill, a skill which produced a number of well-engineered coups. He was immensely proud of his two daughters, but posed as a caricature of the worst type of stern, ferocious Victorian father, a racing Barratt of Wimpole Street! Both girls, who have been most successfully married for some time now, rode quite beautifully. Their father mounted them well and, stood no nonsense from them or their ponies, abusing them for every mistake, but always ready with apparently grudging praise for effort. Jenny, the elder girl, had an excellent jumping pony and another little star to ride sent from an excellent horsewoman from Yorkshire, who has consistently produced top-class show animals.

Generally among larger horses, mares and geldings have little actual brain, but wonderful memories. Across the board, colts and stallions seem to have more intelligence. Ponies, on the other hand, have a double share of brain, but it is frequently naughty and sometimes downright bad. Let me elaborate by way of example: —

Jack Dowdeswell, the bravest of the brave, champion

jockey in his time, was still right at the top of the tree in the jumping world. Despite his somewhat top-heavy build, Jack has always been a fine all-round horseman. He gave his small son Michael, a pony which was far removed from the classy, expensive little numbers which flat race jockeys can afford to give to their children. Like most of our moorland ponies, it was very tough and, if allowed to have its own way, extremely bloody minded.

"It'd been pulling Michael's leg for so long and getting away with it, that it was becoming a real handful," said Jack. "So I decided to teach it a lesson."

With short child (or racing) length stirrup leathers he sat on the pony, flapping the reins and pretending to ride like a little boy for more than an hour. Accordingly, the beast refused to do anything, napped and carried him time and again into trees and bushes, just as it had done with Michael. Then, "When it really thought it had won and was lulled into a sense of security, I suddenly caught hold of it, drew my whip and set about it. I've never known an animal so shocked. Its little eyes popped out of its head and it did just what I told it. It might seem a little unfair, but that pony learnt its lesson and was as good as gold from then on."

This summer Ginger had been schooling both his daughters so successfully that he decided to take them over to the great Dublin Horse Show. Jenny's own pony performed very well indeed, but the other behaved abominably. Before that vast audience of critical horse lovers it refused to take any interest in the proceedings, wouldn't jump a twig and made a complete fool of its rider.

Ginger was understandably furious with the Yorkshire pony. As soon as he got him home, he began schooling him again from scratch; but the pony now resolutely refused to co-operate. He still lolloped around with no interest, stopping at every obstacle. Eventually, completely exasperated, Ginger asked me, "Why the hell don't we dope him?" At that time the racing world was full of dope and rumours about it, but I explained that I had no practical experience of doping horses. Nevertheless, I said that I would have a go.

I got some caffeine from the chemist and worked out the appropriate dose. I arrived at the appointed time and, with help from the family, poured the caffeine down the pony's throat.

"What's going to happen?" asked Ginger.

"The pony should suddenly liven up and take off," I replied expectantly.

So Jenny was loaded on to his back and led out into the paddock where all the schooling show-jumps were and where an audience of family and friends were waiting. We waited with baited breath, everybody growing paler as we anticipated the explosion ... Nothing happened. It was a total anti-climax. Eventually Ginger screamed to Jenny to get off the pony. "I'll ride it myself!"

Jenny jumped off hurrriedly and her father leapt onto the pony's back, determined to teach it a proper lesson just like Jack Dowdeswell. Now we should see something. The master clearly was in no mood to stand any nonsense. But clearly the caffeine had taken longer than expected to be assimilated. As Ginger dug his heels into the pony's sides the little animal suddenly woke up. Without any warning it bucked him firmly onto the ground and trotted back into its box!

Ginger was still seething with rage when we got back to the house. He poured a couple of strong drinks and launched into a tirade against young vets who didn't know their job. When the telephone rang, he barked into it. "It's for you." Without putting his hand over the mouthpiece he added, "Bert Lammin, that farmer near Abingdon. I don't know why the hell he wants you. He'd do better with a grocer's boy!" I ignored the comment and took the phone. Mr Lammin had a mare who was apparently very lame and he wanted me to come over at once. I said I would. When I told Ginger, he said, "I'll take you. You'll probably need my expert knowledge and in any case I'd like to see what sort of a nonsense you can make of this case!" So he got out the old Rolls and off we trundled to the Lammin farm.

Bert was waiting for us when we arrived. He had got the Land Rover out in readiness. Typical of the best products of the area, he was a well-built young farmer, owning some eight hundred acres, with a cherry red face. He loved his shooting and hunting and was fairly successful every spring with his point-to-pointers and hunters-chasers.

We transferred to the Land Rover and were driven up to one of the water meadows. As we scrambled out, Bert took a twelve-bore shotgun from the back of the vehicle. I didn't give it much thought. He would probably go off to shoot some pigeons when we had finished. The mare was a good hunter-chaser who eventually proved the dame of a decent horse that finished third in the Grand National. Ginger held her head while I picked up her foot. To his sardonic amusement I didn't have to look far to make my diagnosis. My searching knife soon discovered a huge abcess. I got to work cleaning the foot and was starting to chop the abscess out when suddenly Bang! right in my ear. The twelve-bore had gone off.

The mare reared up and plunged, knocking Ginger over and kicking me into a heap behind. As I picked myself up I shouted, "What the bloody hell did you do that for? What are you playing at?"

He was quite unperturbed. "Don't worry," he said. "It's all right. I have to take a few shots at the old bull. Otherwise he'll have us."

Then I noticed only a short way away a great big old Friesian bull with a ring in his nose and a wire scar over his face. He was snorting, lowering at us, digging up the ground as he approached with his head down. So Bert fired the second barrel at him and the old bull stopped in his tracks and went back a few paces.

Ginger and I were considerably shaken.

"Do you always do that?" I asked Bert.

"I wouldn't come in this field without the twelve-bore."

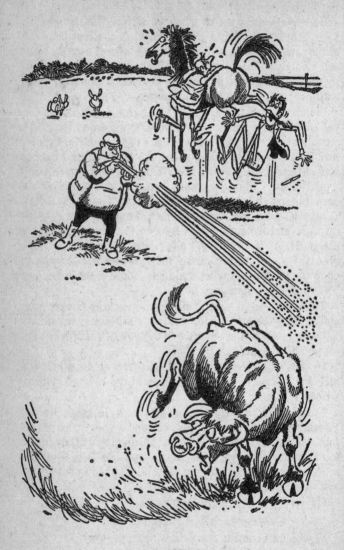

I managed to remove the abcess after this, accompanied by several further interruptions as Bert fired cartridges at his threatening bull. By the time we got back to the farmhouse, Ginger and I badly needed fortifying again!

# LONG DOG

It was just before noon when I drove up to Letcombe Grange. But on this occasion my business was not with the Guv'nor, old George Makepeace.

As I walked into the yard, a loose-box door burst open and a round, light brown figure, clutching a feed-tin, hurtled backwards on to the lawn in the middle, turned a couple of somersaults and collapsed on the grass with arms and legs stretched out like a fat, beached starfish. After a minute the figure came to life again, looked up and shouted, "That's how it happened. Look up! Close the door, boy. You'll let the old girl out again."

I saw two apprentices, who had been watching the demonstration in amazed delight, hurry to obey. At that moment Jack Davies looked round, saw me and scrambled somewhat shamefacedly to his feet, straightening his cap, hitching up his trousers and brushing off his light tan kennel-coat.

"Oh, it's young Mr Dawson. I was just showing them what happened this morning when I went to give old Abigail her breakfast. Caught me right here, sir, in the middle, she did." He clutched his stomach with both hands. "Very lucky it wasn't a bit lower, sir. Then whoosh! She booted me right out of the box!" Before I could stop him, he had turned another backward somersault. Jack was never able to tell a story without demonstrating it. He looked at me with a half smile as I laughed helplessly. Then he shouted, "Get your forks and tidy up that dung-pit, boys, before second lot comes in. We've got serious business to discuss."

When they were out of earshot, he said with a conspiratorial air, "Come into the tackroom, David." He closed the

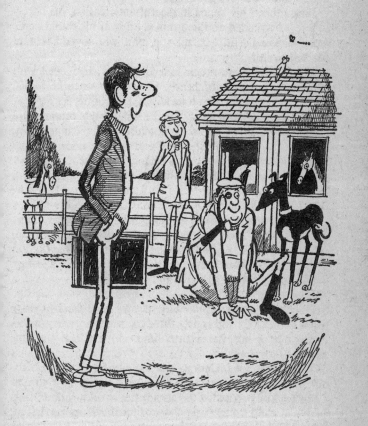

door behind us, sat down, motioned me to the only other chair. After we had lit our pipes, he asked, "Well, have you got one?"

"Yes," I said. "I heard from the track kennels this morning. I think it's a very good one."

Jack rubbed his hands in gleeful anticipation, his happy little eyes wrinkled and he grinned all over his round apple face. A splendid little barrel of a man, who loved beer and sport above all.

The headman, for such indeed he was, had been with George Makepeace for nearly forty years since he joined him as a raw young Welsh jockey just out of his apprenticeship and already too heavy for the flat. Tough, fearless and a fine horseman, he was soon notching up the winners and, before long, was understudying and sharing rides with the stable-jockey, who was British Champion at the time!

Despite the usual ups-and-downs of a jump jockey's life, all went well for several years until the stable had two runners in the Cheltenham Gold Cup. Coming up the hill for the second time, it looked as though the champ might have chosen wrong, Jack was going so far into the lead. Then, galloping at classic speed into the notorious ditch at the top of the hill, his horse never took off, went straight through the bottom, turned right over and buried Jack.

Even with the finest medical treatment that George Makepeace's money could buy, it was three weeks before he was conscious and nearly three months before he was allowed out of hospital with a limp and a severe warning never to race again.

When war came, George was too old for active service, but, as a 1914-18 reservist, managed to join up again as a captain and persuaded the authorities to allow him to take Jack, who had failed every form of 'medical', as his driver-batman. The old trainer's ingenuity did not end there. He wangled a job, with orders to catch deserters, in neutral Southern Ireland. He and Jack caught no deserters, but they enjoyed some wonderful racing and hunting with old friends, made many new ones and established lasting contacts, which enabled George and his new headman to remain near the top of the trainer's list for several years after the war.

It suited both men when age forced the trainer to reduce his string, because Jack's poor shattered bones were none too clever in the cold, damp downland winters. He remained, however, as courageous and cheerful as ever, constantly clowning (which I could see sometimes hurt like hell) with a fund of anecdotes.

Soon after I arrived at Lambourn I had met Jack knocking back pints in the Malt Shovel with a brindle greyhound lying at his feet. We exchanged more delicious draught bitter and, learning that I was the new, obviously green young vet, started talking about his youth in Wales as a professional boy runner, rider of "flapping" ponies at unlicensed race-meetings and trainer of dogs at equally unlicensed greyhound and whippet meetings.

"Pity you can't stop a dog like they used to stop me when my trainer wasn't trying," he complained. "They used to put lead in my spiked running shoes. What a difference when they eventually took the weight out and had a big bet on me!" He chortled into his beer and gratefully put out his tankard for a refill. When I sat down again, he went on; "I learnt how to turn a galloping racehorse over, if all other methods failed, by putting my toe under his elbow and twisting like this. I wouldn't do it now, mind!" He did not do it again that night in the Malt either, because his violently twisted toe upset the table and our beer all over the greyhound.

When order was restored and our tankards were recharged, Jack, quite undismayed, returned to his theme. "Different with dogs now, isn't it, sir? Mind, you can stick chewing gum in their pads and, long as it's not spotted as they are inspected beforehand and put into the traps, that can do the trick. Of course, they could have picked it up on the way round – people are always chewing and spitting these days. But you can't rely on it. You used to be able to put a rubber-band round their toes, but you can't get

117

away with that now." Nostalgia almost had him weeping into the remains of his bitter. This time he gave me the dog's lead while he bought the pints. On his return he lowered his voice. "Trouble with this one is that he never tries nowadays. He's never bloody well 'off', just won't put it in. Used to be a flyer before he went wrong and could be again. I suppose you couldn't help him find his old form, could you, sir?"

In those early days few knew much about the various aspects of doping and most trainers had their own special "tonics" handed down from father to son. They were generally strychnine-based and illegal today. So, full of beer and flushed with youthful enthusiastic liking for this wonderful character, I suggested a tonic mixture for the dog's next appearance at Swindon, which was then an unlicensed track. Unhappily Jack, over-keen as ever, gave the poor dog an overdose, for, no sooner had the brindle dog left his trap, than he collapsed and took some time to recover. I dared not try again and, as he was a proven rogue, he was found a good home in the village. I felt a certain obligation to Jack and, when he learnt that an old college friend of mine was vet to one of the major London tracks, he never lost an opportunity of asking me to find him another good dog.

On licensed tracks a greyhound, which fights (however mildly), plays or otherwise interferes with rival dogs and the course of a race, is disqualified for "turning its head" and warned off for life. It is banned from racing and breeding so, to all intents and purposes, is finished. Thus a dog, which is worth £10,000 today, can be looking for a good home at a maximum figure of £25 tomorrow. This was the kind of dog we were looking for – a brilliant performer, who might regain his form and run his race out true, if he were first allowed to whet his appetite on some good strong live downland hares, which he might never catch by himself, and some live rabbits, which he would.

We had had several false alarms over the next few years, but now, in the Letcombe tack-room, I was able to inform him that a big black greyhound would be arriving at Wan-

118

tage station at 2.30 the next afternoon. Jack asked excitedly, "Will he be addressed to me? How much do I owe you, David?"

"He's all yours and there's nothing to pay. My friend was given the dog after it had been warned off and we've settled the transport between us."

"Clive's letter says he's a very big dog – racing weight seventy-eight pounds." Jack whistled, leaning forward, eyes shining.

I saved the best news to last and said nonchalantly. "Incidentally I hear that you may know the dog. He won a big television race and has appeared on the box several times. He's called Magnetic Hussar."

Jack leapt up, seized my hand and pumped it up and down. His joy knew no bounds. "Of course I know the big black beauty with his white shirt-front and paws. I knew you'd do me proud in the end, boyo. What a dog to own!"

"What are you going to call him, Jack? Even at Swindon he can't go under his own name."

Jack thought out aloud, "Black and White ... Whisky. That's it! We'll call him Whisky – Dawson's Whisky in honour of you."

Despite my pleasure at his gratitude, I demurred slightly. I thought it might be better if a practising local vet was not known to be involved in any way, particularly in view of the last incident, not forgetting that in the fifties, doping was very much in the racing news, hitting the headlines every other day. I thanked Jack for the thought, but said, "Let's just call him Whisky, Jack. It's simpler. Besides what could sound better than 'Mr Jack Davies' Whisky'?"

We got up as we heard second lot coming into the yard. "I'll stand you several doubles on the strength of that, if you'll come down to the Malt tomorrow night. And you can see him, too."

He was as good as his word. I found Jack trying quite unsuccessfully to appear off-hand and conceal his pride in the biggest, most beautiful canine racing machine that I have seen. Straight from London's premier track kennels, his coat shone like ebony. He was so deep through the heart and packed such obvious power in those huge hindquarters. The great, long head with dark brown eyes and smiling patent-leather lips, combined with a tremendous personality, proclaimed a real ruling aristocrat among dogs.

In the next few weeks Jack's relations with the local farmer, Trevor Anderson, became a trifle strained. Suspicion, aroused when the week's supply of meat for his large family, including five beef joints and a big turkey, disappeared from the box by the drive gate where the local butcher's van used to leave it, hardened to certainty when Whisky swooped at 40 mph on the fierce farm cat, which had hitherto terrorised trespassers on his territory, and exhibited his trophy proudly to all. That cost Jack quite a few drinks. But, as he pointed out quite reasonably, the poor fellow hunted by eye and had never seen anything except a stuffed wool hare all his life. How could he know the difference?

Whisky made up for any embarrassment in the finest possible style when he proved strong, fast and agile enough to kill the toughest downland hares single-handed. Full of hope, Jack took his dog to Swindon for the compulsory trials. Whisky did not disappoint him. Even a drink beforehand failed to prevent him from winning by half a track. I was afraid that there would be no chance of a bet in his first race, but at least Jack would have the glory.

In his next trial he repeated the performance and was pronounced fit to race. But the London stewards had not erred in their judgement. Jack was so confident now, that he saw no reason to slip Whisky any more live hares and, in an unofficial run before the big day all Magnetic Hussar's bad habits re-appeared. After running a few yards, he waited for the other dogs, attacked them playfully on the first bend and all the way down the back straight, effectively ruining the trial.

Instead of being sunk in despair, as I had expected when I went to Letcombe to commiserate, Jack had already solved the problem. "What would we do with a brilliant horse, who turned it up, David, me boyo?" he asked. "We'd run him in blinkers. Look what Sam Burke, the saddler, has made for him? We can have a little bet after all." He pulled out the neatest little pair of blinkers – a model of the racehorse version – and fitted them lovingly to Whisky's big, stupid, loving black head. They fitted exactly.

This, I thought, I cannot miss. So on the evening of the race I drove Jack and Whisky to Swindon in my own car.

In the parade before the race Jack wore a white kennel-coat and limped round, leading Whisky, who completely dwarfed and outclassed his opponents, as might be expected. Just before they were due to enter the traps, he fitted the blinkers. Whisky was wearing the black and white striped No. 6 coat and, as the electric hare hurtled round in front, he hurtled from the outside trap, crossed nonchalantly to the inside rail and by half-way it had ceased to be a race. He was obviously coming home alone. Beside me Jack was jumping for joy and shouting his dog home.

Suddenly he stopped, because Whisky had stopped – pulled himself right up, sat down and was busy trying to scratch the blinkers off, oblivious to the other dogs and the shouts of the crowd.

Not knowing whether to laugh or cry, Jack collected the dog, whom he now worshipped, and removed the blinkers. On our way to the nearest pub for a few stiff doubles, he kept his arms round Whisky, buried his face in the black dog's neck and repeated, "You old bugger! You dear silly old bugger! What a pair of stupid buffers we both are!" And there were big tears in his eyes as he looked ruefully at me. "I should have known better, David. At my age I ought to have known better, oughtn't I? Fancy doing that to a beautiful dog, making a fool of him like that. I'm more grateful to you than ever for finding him for me. He's brought a new meaning to my life. We'll buy him a good steak now."

The human members of the party were considerably the worse for wear when we arrived back and I dropped Jack and Whisky at the headman's cottage at Letcombe.

I had to visit the yard the following morning to see a horse for George Makepeace. Whisky was romping about in great form, but, when his master appeared, I saw that he was attempting to keep his cap covering a black eye.

"Run into a box door or a lamp-post?" I asked.

Jack became dramatic. "When I put the dog to bed last night," he said, "I took off my shoes and started to climb the stairs to bed. Not a sound I made. But I slipped and there at the top of the stairs was a great white ghost gazing down at me. As I got near, she shouted, 'You're not coming up here tonight, you drunken fool, Jack Davies. You can sleep with your dog.' With that the ghost swings a powerful right to my left eye and I go backwards down the stairs all the way to the bottom. Boom! Boom! Boom! Boom! Boom!" With each boom he bounced on his back on the grass.

After I had treated the horse and talked to George, I looked back as I left the yard. There in the middle sat Jack with his black dog lying adoringly beside him, surrounded by hysterical stable-lads.

Their black-eyed headman was in contortions as he tried to get his right foot high enough to scratch his face, while he told a story, which would, I knew, last him for the rest of his life.

# A CLAIM FOILED

INSURANCE brings out the best and also the worst in horse owners. I had two cases in about ten days, one of which emphasised Man's cupidity and the other the more generous side of Man's make-up.

The first concerned John Cobbold, a very big, rich farmer from down in the Vale. He was a bluff, heavy, hard-riding man in his sixties. I knew him well from various excursions I had made into the hunting field. He was a fearless horseman, with little or no regard for his animals. I had seen him literally ride a horse into the ground, when it was so tired from a long day in heavy plough, that it could not get one foot in front of the other.

On this particular occasion, after weeks of heavy rain, we were hunting a fresh fox through a part of the country which was well supplied with hunt fences, but was quite bottomless. There were four of us on our own as we galloped across a meadow towards the Military College of Science at Shrivenham. In the corner of the field was a stile, surrounded by ground which had been well poached by cattle. Willy Fairbairn, the young amateur whip, was in front, and he set sail for the stile. He had turned to have a second try, when Cobbold thundered up on his old brown heavyweight hunter. "Get out of the bloody way, and let those that can go have a bit of daylight," he roared at Willy. Jacob was certainly one of the safest jumpers in the country, and, true as ever, he stood off and flew the stile. I was about to follow his lead, when I saw the rider in front being decanted from the saddle with some force. The big horse had gone down on his nose, but I could see that he had regained his balance and was making off across the next field.

"Keep down, sir," I yelled. "I think I can clear you."

With which kindly warning, I aimed my mount, a retired steeplechaser, at the fence. Even as I was in the air, Cobbold started to rise to his feet, shouting a warning about staying where I was. Too late, I saw to my horror that there was a deep ditch on the landing side, which was almost filled with water. My horse reached out and touched down beyond the edge of the water, but his hind feet scrabbled for a non-existent foothold and he subsided in a skidding heap. I sprawled over, grabbing at tufts of long grass as I went, trying to keep myself out of the water and ended up in an undignified heap alongside the irate farmer. "You damn fool, I told you to wait," he spluttered.

"Sorry about that," I gasped. "But for God's sake keep down! Here comes Mrs Barnet." No sooner said, than there was a splintering crash as her little horse missed his take-off, shattered the top of the stile, and landed in a flurry of feet and legs alongside us. Like the other two, the mare scrambled up and made off towards the sound of the hounds, leaving her rider to join our muddied and winded little gathering.

After scraping some of the glutinous mud off my face and hands, I went over to Mrs Barnet. She was a sad sight. Her immaculate coat and breeches had suffered the same fate as her carefully applied make-up. She was gasping in that painful manner that you do when winded, struggling to force air into your lungs and wondering whether you will ever succeed again. After a couple of minutes she shook herself, like a spaniel coming out of a brook, and gave a watery smile, announcing that she was going to live. By this time, Cobbold had got to his feet and was poking about in the mud, muttering obscenities. When I saw that my companions were undamaged, I set off in pursuit of the horses, and found they had been thwarted at the top of the field by a large iron gate, which was thankfully firmly closed. As I got near, I managed to seize the reins of Mr Cobbold's hunter, and was just about to grab the little mare, when my own horse whipped round and shoved her away. She shot back down along the hedge. However I succeeded in clutching the rein of my own horse before he followed his female acquaintance. Pulling him to a standstill, I climbed into the saddle, and trotted back to the stile with the big hunter in tow. Then I noticed that he was going very short on his off foreleg.

I got back to his owner, who was still engaged in sifting through the muddy pool. Mrs Barnet had captured her own horse, as it cantered back to the others.

"I caught your horse, sir, but I'm afraid he is too lame to go with," I said, proffering the reins to the farmer.

"Never mind about the bloody horse. Get off and help me find my blasted teeth," he growled. So that was what he was combing the ground for. Telling the lady of the party to push on to the hunt, I slid off my horse to join the search. Before long my foot revealed the missing dentures, grinning up at me from their watery hiding place. "There they are," I said.

The bold rider bent down to recapture his falsies, but, at the same moment, his horse spun round and put a large soup-plate foot straight on top of them.

"You careless sod," he swore, as he picked up the teeth, now decidedly the worse for wear. This was too much and, passing over his horse with the advice that he take him straight home, I trotted off to the gate, rejoined the field in the college grounds, and had to put up with various rude comments about choosing a dry ditch if I wanted to disturb Mary Barnet's attire. I told the Master about John Cobbold's misfortune, but, just as a crowd was gathering to hear the tale of the teeth, there was a holloa from the far side of the covert, and we all set off again.

An hour later, when I was hacking back to my horse-box, I met half a dozen riders trotting down the road. To my amazement, in among them was Cobbold, whose poor horse was very lame by now. "For Heaven's sake, take that poor fellow home," I shouted as he passed.

"When I want your lousy advice, I'll ask for it and no doubt pay heavily for it too," he snarled. "I haven't forgotten how you deliberately broke my plate for me."

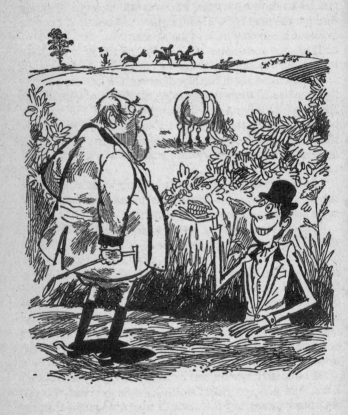

Fuming at his last remark, I loaded up and made for Lambourn. At a party later that evening I saw some of the hunting farmers who were still embellishing the story of our disasters at the stile. They were full of helpful advice as to what I should tell Mr Cobbold to do with his false teeth – he was by no means the most popular man in the district. But I told them I was far too worried about poor Jacob.

Two days later, I looked at the day book in the surgery and saw that there was a message for me to call at Mr Cobbold's to see a lame horse. Not in the least surprised at the request, I visited his farm that afternoon. I found my client in the stable yard abusing Janet, the poor girl who looked after his four hunters. As he heard my footsteps, he turned round and gave me a wintry smile. "Ah, Dawson, that horse which fell on Saturday is still lame. You'd better see what is wrong with him, because I want him this Saturday."

I noticed that he was once again equipped with a shining set of dentures, and remarked that I was glad that he had managed to get them repaired.

"Repaired be damned. I had to get a new set. I have a good mind to set the cost off against your bill."

As there was no point in prolonging the argument over the disintegration of the original set, I went into Jacob's box. The unfortunate horse was resting his off fore, which was greatly swollen by this time. He was clearly in considerable pain and, no doubt, the continued work after his fall had aggravated the trouble more than a little. Picking up the leg, I ran my fingers down the tendons. Without a shadow of a doubt he had severely strained his tendons from the knee all the way down to the fetlock. Looking up at the owner, I said, "I'm very sorry Mr Cobbold, but he will certainly not be fit to hunt again this season. If we rest him and then fire his legs in a month's time, he should be all right for the odd day next year."

Cobbold was obviously annoyed at my prognosis, although from his next remark it was not unexpected. "Now then, he is insured for £750. If you can give me a certificate to say that he will not come right, I can claim for him and have him put down."

This line of reasoning was not unknown and, in his case, I thought it typical of his attitude to his horses. Still, I knew that he had hunted Jacob for the past five seasons, and claimed that he was the best hunter he had ever ridden. It seemed churlish treatment at best to decide to shoot the poor horse, rather than treat and rest him. Moreover I was fairly sure that his insurance policy only covered cases of humane destruction where the animal was in such pain that he would never recover. This was obviously not such a case, because a few poultices would take away the pain, and treatment would render him sound enough for light hunting if nothing more. I explained the position to the owner, who waved my reasoning aside, answering that he would get a second opinion. "Anyway," he went on, "you don't have to say that it's a sprained tendon. Tell the insurance people that he has broken a bone in his joint. I'll send him to the kennels tomorrow, and you write out a piece of paper stating that you recommend his destruction."

It seemed that the best line was to advise him to contact his insurance company, tell them the story and ask them to give me a ring. He grudgingly agreed to this, and went off to phone. As I turned to go the girl groom caught my arm. "Mr Dawson," she said. "I shouldn't really tell you, but I wanted to put on a poultice when he came home. Mr Cobbold wouldn't let me, because he said the horse would never be any more use, and he wanted him to look as bad as possible before you came to see him. I've been bathing his leg in warm water, when Mr Cobbold was out at market, but it doesn't seem to have done much good."

I assured her that I was not blaming her at all and that I did not think her employer had a cat's chance in hell of collection off the company.

That evening a friend, who was employed as a veterinary adviser for Lloyds' insurance groups rang me. I told him what I knew of the case, that the horse was pretty bad, but that I thought he would come sound with time. He asked if

I was prepared to say that his injury was such that he would never be out of pain, and, when I answered that I would certainly not do that, he thanked me and said he would inform the principals that there was no justifiable claim.

The following evening I was boiling up my instruments in the surgery when the phone rang. I answered and a familiar voice asked for Mr Grill urgently. I ran through to the office and found the senior partner. I told him that Mr Cobbold wanted to speak to him. I watched him talk, and asked him as soon as he put down the phone what he had had to say.

"He wants me to go straight away and see a horse which he thinks should be destroyed because it is in terrible pain."

I told him the outline of the story and wished him luck.

The next morning I could hardly wait to get to the surgery to hear how my employer had got on the previous evening.

"I shot the horse," said Eric. "He was unable to take any weight on his leg and the tendons were completely ruptured."

I was stunned. How on earth had he deteriorated to that extent in a day? I had to go past the stables that afternoon and I called in to have a word with the groom. I found the cowman in the yard and asked for Janet.

"Sweet on her are you?" he leered – just the sort of man who would work for Cobbold. I pressed him to tell me where she was.

"I've no idea. She took off last night and said she would never come back and she didn't care whether the boss gave her a reference or not."

Puzzled by the turn of events, I returned to Lambourn in the evening. I had only been in about five minutes when Jim called me to the phone. It was Janet. "I'm ringing from Swindon," she said. "I couldn't make up my mind whether I should tell you or not, but I thought you should know that Mr Cobbold took that horse out yesterday morning and lunged him for an hour. When I complained, he told me to shut up and that now the vets would have to agree to put the horse down. I was so upset that I walked out and didn't even wait for my week's pay." She sounded so tearful on the phone that I asked if she had another job in view. She said that she was staying with her sister-in-law and would go to the labour exchange tomorrow. I remembered that I had been asked by another client if I knew where there was a good groom for some polo-ponies, so I gave her the address. In return, I told her that she must be prepared to let me have a letter confirming exactly what her boss had done. She took a bit of persuading but the thought of her late charge being summarily sent to the kennels was too strong, and she agreed.

I saw Mr Grill and told him what I had learned. He was furious and said he would tell Cobbold that he would certainly not give him a certificate. To all our surprise, although he blustered, that gentleman, did not pursue the matter. Not surprisingly, we lost a client. But, as Jim remarked, there were enough bad bastards in the world without us having to work for them. He followed this with one of his notorious winks. "David, my boy, you'd better make sure that you never try to jump upsides him at a fence in future. He's sure to do you."

In fact, Mr Cobbold was never to speak to me again. He studiously avoided me out hunting and, if we ever met, he managed to look straight past me. I certainly never tried to renew our unhappy acquaintance.

# A CLAIM AVOIDED

THE second insurance problem was very different from that involving John Cobbold. It concerned an extremely valuable horse which was trained by William Green.

I was getting dressed to go to a hunt dance with Jeannie when the phone pealed its imperious summons. I had told Jim that I would be off duty that evening, but most of my clients, including William, had adopted the habit of ringing me at home. This was a mixed blessing in that it occasionally interrupted my love life, but, on the whole, I much preferred to have this direct contact with clients who were also my friends. I answered the phone while struggling to knot my bow-tie.

"David," William began in a worried voice. "I'm not at all happy about that good colt of mine, which I bought at the Houghton Sales. He looks very dull and miserable tonight, and he's not touched his evening feed."

I sighed. Undoubtedly our dance was going to be delayed. I knew that this particular horse was the apple of William's eye, and that he would not have bothered me unless he was really worried. "Has he got a temperature?" I asked.

The trainer assured me that his temperature was only half a degree above normal, but could I possibly look in on my way to the party? Remembering that I had told him I was going to take Jeannie out that night, I said that I would pick her up and come that way to have a quick look at the colt.

Putting the receiver down, I grabbed my jacket and went out to the car. I arrived at Jeannie's cottage, and went in to break the news that we were going to make a slight detour on our way.

"David, you're impossible," she said, wrinkling her nose

131

in an irresistible way. "Why can't you forget about your work for one evening? Surely there is someone else to go and see the animal? I suppose it's about twenty miles in the wrong direction."

I assured her that it was only just out of our way. In fact it was only nineteen miles in completely the opposite direction to the dance. I apologised and promised that it would only take five minutes, but that it was important that we have a look at the horse.

With her auburn hair and super figure accentuated by the long, tight-fitting sapphire blue dress, I was tempted to let William make his own arrangements for that evening. However my conscience won, as it was to do so many times in later years, to the frustrated fury of my future wife and family. It was not entirely a question of a Florence Nightingale approach to my profession, but a mixture of worry for my friends' charges, combined, I suppose, with a slight conceit that they preferred my advice to that of any of my colleagues.

I persuaded the lovely Jeannie into the car with a pressing embrace and a promise of an uninterrupted evening when we reached the festivities. Muttering about how she would have been better off accepting an invitation from Johnny English, an amateur jockey who vied with me for her favours, she climbed into the front seat. I drove like a demon, which had the satisfactory effect of causing my companion to clutch my knee in what I chose to believe was a loving embrace but, was more like real terror.

We arrived at the training stable on the downs to be met by William, standing in the middle of the yard. "David, it is good of you to come. I'm not sure whether I've called you out on a wild goose chase or not." He smiled ruefully as I got out. "He doesn't look too bad, but I can't think why he isn't eating, and I'd planned to give him another run at Ascot next week." Seeing Jeannie in the passenger seat, he went round to her door and asked if she wanted to come and see the horse.

"If you think I've put on my glad rags just to hold a wake

132

at the bedside of your wretched horse, Willy, you're mistaken. You can have David for five minutes. After, I am claiming him back for the rest of the night," she replied acidly.

It looked as though unless I complied with her wishes, she might well drive herself to the dance and leave me to stew. So I took the hint, picked up my stethoscope and hurried off to the patient.

William went on ahead to get a headcollar, while I stood by the box door to watch the colt. He was a fine big chestnut with large bold eyes set in an intelligent face, which typified a class horse. I knew him well, since every time I had been to the yard for the past six months, I had been sent over to look at him. He had raced for the first time about a fortnight before, and had lived up to all expectations by cantering home an easy winner in a good two-year-old race at Salisbury.

As I stood watching the colt, I could see why William was worried. He clearly was not his usual cheeky self; he displayed no interest when I opened the door, but stayed in the middle of his box, with his head held listlessly and his eyes half closed. We put the headcollar on him, and I took his temperature – still just above normal. His pulse and his respiration were normal but, listening through the stethoscope, I could hear some strange rumblings and squeakings in his belly. His eyelids and mouth seemed to be a nice salmon pink colour, which did not indicate any serious trouble. Standing back, I debated what line of treatment to advise, which would ensure that both Trolly (the colt's stable name, his official name being Troilus) and William had a peaceful night's rest.

"It looks as though he's got a tummy upset. I don't suppose it's much, but we'd better be on the safe side and give him a dose of kaolin and chalk to settle his insides."

"O.K. But isn't that going to muck up your smart trousers?"

Assuring him with misplaced confidence that it would only take a minute and that my smock would preserve my

133

finery, I went to get my stomach tube and the necessary medicine.

I told Jeannie what was happening and promised to be no more than five minutes.

"I know you, David," she answered with a sigh. "I'll come and hold the beast for you, and make sure you hurry up." Despite my protests that William and I could manage, she followed me up the path. William had collected a bucket of warm water and a bridle to put on the horse. "Hello Jeannie," he said abstractedly, as she walked up. "You can hold his head and then I can work the pump for David."

"And what about my evening dress?" she snapped. "You men are all the same. You're so involved with your damned horses that you never notice anything else."

Willy apologised hastily and said he would find a coat in the tack room for her.

By the time he came back I was ready to dose the patient. I carried the bucket with its mixture of white medicaments into the box and looked up to find an extraordinary apparition holding the horse. Willy had equipped Jeannie with an outsize mac, which hung like a collapsed tent from her shoulders, and, worse still, had covered her head with a brand new pair of blinkers.

"Doesn't she look attractive? Pity the ear holes are too far apart or we could have fitted them over her eyes and you could go on to your dance with Jeannie dressed as a highwayman."

"I don't think that it's at all funny," she said in a muffled voice, as the straps of the hood caught under her chin. "Do get on David, or I'll go home and you can dance on your own – if you ever succeed in getting there." I stifled my laughter at the sight of my assistant. I could see the danger signs of Jeannie's Irish temper welling up.

It is a common-place operation in horse practice to administer medicine by a stomach-tube. Although it looks a painful procedure, the vast majority of horses will swallow a tube with no bother at all. The tricky part is to persuade the end of the tube to pass down the gullet and not into the windpipe. Occasionally it seems to develop a determination of its own to investigate the lower reaches of the lungs. Perhaps it was because I was trying to hurry or perhaps just because the tube itself decided to be awkward, after four attempts, I still had not managed to slide it down the gullet. I knew that my lady friend was now rapidly going off both the horse and, worse still, me.

I withdrew the end of the tube from his throat. Suddenly calamity struck. As the tube flicked back down his nostril, Trolly coughed, and my vision was obscured by a shower of blood. The great hazard of the operation is the risk of breaking one of the many small blood vessels in the back of the nose. On the average it happened to me about once in every two hundred horses. Once the bleeding starts, it keeps on in a steady stream for a couple of minutes. The presence of fluid in the horse's throat stimulates his cough reflex and that, in turn, ensures that the operator and attendants get liberally painted in red. In fact, within seconds it looked as though all three of us had been attacked by a madman with a paint spray. Jeannie gave a shout of anguish as her blinkers dropped over her face. William jumped forward to her assistance, and at that moment the tube slid effortlessly down the gullet as though it was satisfied with its effects and had decided at last to co-operate.

"Sorry about that," I apologised. "Hold on a minute now, and we can pump in the medicine and get off."

Once again I had under-estimated the importance which women place on their appearance for a party.

"If you think I'm going to a bloody dance like this, you're more stupid than you look," she said, her temper definitely getting the better of her. "You can put your things back in the car and take me straight home."

I washed off the tube and pump, cleaned up the unfortunate horse's face as best I could and went to help Jeannie out of her so-called protective clothing. Alas, it had not been protective enough, and her dress and face were spattered with red splodges. William was fussing round apologetically. He suggested that we have a drink in his house and Jeannie could easily repair the damage in the bathroom. His offer was scornfully dismissed, as she made for the car, got in and firmly slammed the door.

"Don't worry, William, it was all my fault. I'll go home and let her sort herself out," I said more optimistically than I felt. "Anyway, Trolly has stopped bleeding and kaolin should ease his stomach. I'll call in tomorrow morning and see how he is."

We drove home in a chilled silence, broken only by the occasional sniff from my companion. I could not tell in the dark whether this meant tears or temper, but when I suggested turning up the road to my place, I quickly understood that it was the latter. "You can take me straight to my cottage, and you needn't bother to wait. I should have realised before that I'm only a poor second to your beloved horses."

I returned to my patient the next morning only to find that he was still far from well. The trainer asked what joy I had had in pacifying Jeannie, and I told him that I had decided to remain a bachelor for life. Brushing aside his sympathies, which were slightly falsified by his amusement at the thought of the poor girl blinkered and blood bespattered, I went to see the colt. He was definitely worse. His temperature had risen, and there were ominous sounds of increased activity in his abdominal cavity. Worse, he was starting to have diarrhoea, and his eyes showed all the indications of a general dehydration.

"I'm afraid he's caught some nasty bug, which has affected his whole digestive system. I'll give him some fluid straight into his bloodstream and we'd better get him started on a course of something to try and kill the germ."

William looked apprehensive. "Are you going to put the tube down him again?"

"I don't think we need rush it at the moment but, if he gets worse then we'll have to try again."

I returned in the evening to find that the diarrhoea was more pronounced and that Trolly had still eaten nothing. Taking my courage in both hands, I summoned the head lad and mixed up a second concoction to try and bind up his inflamed intestines. This time the tube went down first time with no bother. The head man grinned and said that he had heard that I had trouble last night. He started to pull my leg about not having my mind on the job, when I broke in and asked if the boss was about. Apparently he had gone off to see an owner, but had left a message saying he would ring me when he got home.

William phoned after dinner to see what I thought about the colt. I explained that I was getting worried about him. I suggested that he should tell the owner that all was not well and ask if the horse was insured. The request had its usual effect of instilling alarm into the trainer, who immediately imagined the worst. I tried to reassure William but I knew he could tell that I was more worried than I let on. I told him to call me first thing in the morning, and then decided to ring Jeannie.

I was answered by her friend, who sounded evasive when I asked to speak to the love of my life. "David," she answered," I don't know what happened between you two last night, but she was in a filthy mood this morning and told me not to mention your name. She's gone out to see Johnny tonight. I don't know when she'll be back. Shall I get her to give you a ring?"

I decided to let things simmer down, thanked her and told her I would leave it for a few days. Things did not look too bright – I was in danger of losing my best patient and also my girl. I poured out a strong whisky and switched on the radio, only to hear some man talking earnestly about the dangers of alcohol. That was all I needed, so I switched him off and went to bed.

The phone rang at half past six. It was William, "I'm not happy about Trolly. He's scouring like fun, and he's lost nearly a hundred-weight during the night. By the way, he is insured – the owner stepped it up to £45,000 after he won at Salisbury."

"That decides it," I answered. "Put him straight into a horse-box and send him into our hospital, where we can keep an eye on him." William agreed and said he would send him over in his own box after first lot.

I rang Jim to warn him that Trolly would be arriving, and sat down over breakfast to think what I could do to arrest the obviously deteriorating situation. I was horrified to see the poor horse when I reached Lambourn. He had indeed lost weight, his face was drawn and his ribs were showing. It was hard to realise that he had looked a picture of a racehorse only some forty-eight hours before. I filled him up with more drugs and gave an intra-venous drip during the morning, then I went off on my rounds. By that evening the horse was becoming weak and he would lean up against the wall for preference. The insurance company had telephoned during the afternoon and said that their veterinary adviser would call the next day to see the horse.

He was no better in the morning and, when the vet came down from London, he held out little hope and offered no further advice as to how to treat the horse. He agreed with me that there was no chance of his surviving unless we could stop the diarrhoea within the next couple of days. "If he gets down and can't get up, I should put him out of his misery," he advised as he left.

For the next two days Trolly steadily lost ground, despite all our efforts. I was sitting in the surgery with Jim when I suddenly had an idea. "Come on, Jim," I said. "We'll have one last go at that horse. Go and pick up some droppings from one of the other horses in the yard, and mix them in a bucket of water. Then pour the contents through a stable rubber, and we'll tip the fluid down Trolly."

Jim looked at me as though I had finally taken leave of my senses. I explained that I just remembered an old vet I had known, who used to take a piece of chewed footstuff from a cow and put it down a calf's throat to stop it scouring. The theory was that, if one could establish some of the normal bacteria which live in the gut back into the inflamed intestine, they would allay the infection.

Jim came out with a half bucketful of the unattractive mixture, and I pumped it down the colt, who was now emaciated and hardly able to stand. "Well, that's it, Jim. If that doesn't work, I'm beat."

"Funny sort of treatment," he snorted. "I thought you young chaps were supposed to be all full of science and drugs with long names."

"We will just have to wait and see. It doesn't look as though modern science has done too much for this one."

Next morning I hurried to see my patient. To my intense disappointment, he was no better. It did not seem that he was scouring so much, but he was desperately weak, still off his food and completely disinterested in everything. His blood count was the same as on the previous day, which indicated that he was still markedly dehydrated. Thoroughly depressed, I went into the office to ring William. "I am afraid we've done no good with your horse. I really feel it would be kinder to stop him suffering any more."

He replied that he would leave it to me to make the final decision.

I waited until Mr Grill came into the yard, and asked him to go and see what he thought about our patient's condition. He came back and confirmed my thoughts. I hung about for the next hour, making excuses to myself for putting off the moment of decision. Finally I could dodge it no longer, picked up my gun and went round to the stables. Jim had offered to help, but I felt that I would rather do the deed on my own. When I pushed open the door, I saw Trolly propped against the far wall. I went up behind him to move him over, and, as I put a hand on his quarters, he picked up his hind leg and half kicked in my direction. I went to his head to pull him round and, for the first time for days, he put back his ears and tried to bite me. As I caught hold of his headcollar, he grabbed a mouthful of hay from the haynet, as if to say, "Let me have one last bit of food."

It was too much for me. It was as if he knew what I had come to do, and was making a determined effort to resist.

I put the gun back in my pocket, and returned to the surgery. "What happened, old boy?" asked Jim. "I never heard the shot."

"No, I couldn't bring myself to do it. I think I'll leave him until this evening. But I definitely shan't let him go through another night."

Miserably I set off on the day's round. I managed to prolong my calls so that it was half-past-six when I returned to Lambourn. As I pulled up, Billy looked round the door with a broad grin. "You'd better go and see your horse, David, but mind he doesn't eat you."

I hurried round to the loose box. Even before I looked over the door, I could hear a steady munching sound. Sure enough there was my patient tucking into a small heap of cut grass. Over-joyed, I went in, and Trolly put back his ears and turned his quarters threateningly towards me.

"O.K. old boy. I won't worry you. You have a lot of eating to catch up with." As I turned to come out, I saw Jim and Billy laughing over the door. "That old chap deserves to live, David. He did his best to tell you to clear off this morning, and since then he's hardly stopped eating."

"It looks as though the old-fashioned treatment has still got its place," I laughed. "But mind you don't give him too much to eat or he'll be right back were he started."

William rang when I got home. "Did you manage to get any news from the post-mortem examination on the colt?"

"Post-mortem, be damned! The horse is nearly fit enough to run again now." I told him the story much to his delight. We agreed that, if all went well, Trolly would go to a stud farm in a few days to recuperate.

It took the horse about three months to regain his former condition, and in the late autumn, I went to William's yard to greet Trolly on his arrival home. He was welcomed as if he had just won the Derby, and clearly he thoroughly enjoyed being the centre of attention. When he was safely into his old box, I retired to drink his health with the trainer.

"Well, thank you, David, for all you've done for Trolly. By the way has Jeannie ever forgiven you for ruining her evening?"

I revealed that that had been the end of a beautiful friendship, but that I had realised she was never cut out to be a vet's wife. She just did not have that blend of complete self-lessness and eternal patience, which marks all the long-suffering spouses of my colleagues. She quite reasonably considered that, on certain occasions, she should have priority over the four-legged creatures.

Trolly went back into training after Christmas and one day in March, William asked me to come up on the gallops with him to listen to a horse. We stood together as three or four cantered past us. One came by making a loud roaring noise as he cantered.

"My God, that's Trolly, isn't it?"

Ruefully William agreed. He explained that he had been worried about his wind since he first cantered a month before. It seemed that his near brush with death had left a permanent mark.

"What do we do now?" I asked. "Are we going to Hob-day him?"

William looked at me, and said, "I think he's suffered enough, don't you? I've told the owner, and he's agreed that I should try and sell him abroad as a stallion. He's beauti-fully bred and, after all, he is a winner of his only race." This was certainly a satisfactory decision from Trolly's view-point.

"How much will you be able to get for him?"

William told me that he had already been offered £15,000 by one of the agencies who were prepared to place him, even though his wind was not right.

Some months later I met the owner in William's yard. He thanked me for all that we had done for Trolly. I pointed out that, in fact, I had cost him £30,000 since I could quite justifiably have destroyed him with the insurance company's blessing. By treating his horse, I had left him with an un-sound animal worth a third of his previous value. He roared with laughter. "That horse gives me more pleasure there, looking out over his box door, than any amount of money would. I would rather keep him at home as a pet than have to destroy him. But I guess he'll be a whole lot happier

141

abroad with his wives than watching me practise my putting on the lawn."

As I said at the beginning – this attitude is a world apart from my hunter client's and, thank Heavens, it is not an altogether unique one.

# THE SLEEPING BAKER

SOME weeks after my escapade with Trolly, Billy asked me to see a lame mare for him at the Cliftons'. She was a show-hack, who had been lame on her near fore for over a month. Billy said that he had been over her with a fine toothcomb but just could not find the root of the trouble. He had suspected a bruise in the sole of the hoof since she flinched when he applied any pressure there. However, numerous poultices had failed to make any significant improvement. The Cliftons were beginning to get impatient, as they were missing an increasingly long period of the showing season. The patient was a part-bred Arab of uncertain temperament. Billy warned me that she was quite likely either to bite me or to direct a well-aimed cow kick at me.

Ruminating over the eccentricities of horses in general and Billy's patients in particular, I drove off to see the man-eater. Billy was short and stout and none too nimble on his feet, which tended to make him an easy target for his more disgruntled patients. Freckle-faced with a mop of unruly red hair, he presented the world with a slightly puzzled expression. This in fact was a delusion, since he was a determined man and attacked any task like a terrier. So much so that he often managed to alarm both the animal and its owner. We once had to rescue him from a large, infuriated boar, which was enjoying a three day stay in the hospital. Quite why it was there, and what it was being treated for, I was never sure. However the bold Billy went into its loosebox to catch it one morning. Deciding that its ears presented the best hand holds, he straddled the creature with his legs and seized an ear in each hand. What ensued sounded like a fair replica of a bucking bronco display, from which the boar emerged the victor. Billy was flung to the straw, and the out-raged pig had turned to the attack. Summoned by his cries, we had rushed to find him leaping around the box like a bull-fighter. We were afraid to open the door in case the patient escaped and caused havoc in the village, so we advised our young colleague to get up into the manger and then climb over the partition into the next box. Alas, we had over-estimated the strength of the manger bolts; or perhaps we had seriously under-estimated Billy's weight. At any rate both Bill and manger descended in a heap at the boar's feet. At this fortuitous moment Paddy Healey arrived with a lunging rein in his hand. We threw this to the beleaguered young vet, who, after a further ballet routine around the box, managed to lasso his opponent and make his escape. From the similarity between this adventure and those in Jim's favourite western films, he not unnaturally earned the nickname of Billy the Kid. Never at a loss to capitalise on a humorous situation, he promptly went off and bought himself a fine pair of leather chaps. Despite all our protests that he looked more like Mickey Rooney trying to look like Gregory Peck, he insisted on wearing them for his rounds. It was only when an over-eager collie on one of the farms mistook him for an errant bullock and tore one leg clean off, that he reverted to more normal gear.

Bringing my mind back to the immediate problem, I considered the likely causes of my new patient's lameness. I knew that the Clifton family were pretty knowledgeable about horses. They would have eliminated all the obvious things like strained tendons, splints and windgalls before they summoned Billy in the first place. I had known them vaguely for many years, having envied their adroitness in shows and gymkhanas from my school days. Jack Clifton was a farmer of some four hundred acres, high on the Downs above Letcombe Regis. He fought a losing battle with his wife and their two daughters to keep the number of horses and ponies within measurable numbers. Before the days of narrow specialisation, the daughters, Ann and Sarah, showed hunters and hacks and usually had at least one show-jumper. As I got out of the car, a flurry of dogs ran at me.

"Don't touch the spaniel," warned Ann, who was the

elder of the two. Tall and blonde with classical features, she would have been at home among the pages of *Vogue*. "You can't trust that old brute. He belongs to my father and nobody else can handle him." She laughed. "You must have come up to see Merry Queen, I'll give Sarah a shout, as she's her mare." She ran off into the cowshed. Joan Clifton was proud of her herd of Jersey cows, which she and her daughters hand-milked at the strangest hours, depending on their departure and return from horse shows. Despite their erratic routine, the cows regularly ranked high in the county lists for their milk yields.

I walked over to the door, and had to jump back as Sarah ran out and nearly knocked me over. "Gosh, I am sorry," she said breathlessly. "I didn't hear the car. Hold on a second and I'll get a bridle for Merry."

Sarah was also tall, but with darker hair, cut in a fierce-looking fringe. She had a detached expression which, until one knew her better, gave the impression of disinterest. However, when she smiled, her whole face lit up with impish merriment. Both girls looked as though they flung their clothes on at random. They obviously followed the example set by their mother, Joan Clifton, who followed Sarah out of the cowshed. She wore an old blue skirt, held together by a large blue nappy-pin, a thick sweater with one arm just hanging together as if by will power, and a well worn Jaqmar scarf on her head. "Come on girls. Don't keep David waiting. Get Daddy to finish the milking, Ann, and I'll hurry Sarah up." She bustled on, pushing the dogs out of the way. "I am glad you could come. I don't think that the little fat boy could find what is wrong with Merry. It's so aggravating, because she won with her at Richmond and we were hoping to take her to the White City for the International."

Mrs Clifton hurried into the tack room, still shouting for Sarah to hurry. She came out again immediately. "Where has that silly girl got to? She's quite likely to have picked up a book and started reading it."

"I'm here, Mummy," came a shout from a stable at the

145

end of a long row of converted calf pens. We went along to join her. Sarah was holding a bold quality mare, a bright chestnut with a large white blaze. Even in the box she gave that imperious look of a mare who expects to be treated like a lady. Telling Sarah to trot her out, I moved back and nearly fell over Mrs Clifton, who was peering over my shoulder. I apologised, but she brushed my remarks aside and urged her daughter to hurry. This was obviously the trade mark of Joan Clifton's life. It was there to be lived with full enjoyment and great impatience. When I mentioned this to Sarah she laughed and told me that I should see her mother when they were in a hurry to leave a horse show. It was like taking a pound note from a Scotsman to winkle her away from all her friends and their show talk.

Sarah trotted the mare up the yard, and I did notice that she was appreciably lame on her near fore although, in all honesty, I found myself more interested in watching how Sarah moved. I was glad to see that she was quite sound and remarkably attractive. I decided that I might be very grateful to Billy for getting me to call at the Cliftons'. I dragged my thoughts back to the mare and followed her into the box and bent to pick up her foot. "I gather she doesn't like vets much," I said nervously.

"Well, she's all right usually, but she did have a go at Mr Foster the other day," Sarah reassured me.

I felt all down the leg, and, as I had suspected, there was nothing unusual there. I went round her foot with the hoof testers without eliciting any undue signs of pain. Her shoes were pressing into her heels where her foot had grown. Seeing me looking at the shoe, Mrs Clifton explained that they had been waiting for the blacksmith for three weeks, but he had been off sick. So I volunteered to remove the shoe – an operation which always showed me up in a bad light when compared with a proper farrier. My buffer never seemed to be sharp enough to get under the clinches, and the pinchers always managed to remove a piece of horn in addition to the shoe – a clear case of a bad workman determinedly blaming his tools. Still, I cleaned out the foot with my knife and began to unearth a deep powder-filled hole at the toe.

"It looks as though we may have found the cause of the pain," I said, looking round at Sarah, who was craning over my back to see what I was doing. To my surprise, I felt an inexplicable thrill run down my spine as I felt her arm brush my back. I quickly returned to my excavating work and pared out an area around the toe, which ran up a good inch inside the outer wall. Ferreting about in the depths of the cavity, I suddenly touched a sensitive area, and the mare jumped up in the air. Hanging on to her foot, I was thrown violently against the wall, while Sarah was knocked into the corner by Merry's head.

"Are you O.K.?" I said, as the wind returned to my lungs.

"I'm perfectly all right," she grinned. "You did well to hang on to her leg."

Encouraged by this praise, I had a closer look at the hoof. What had upset the mare was my opening a deep-seated abscess in the wall of the hoof. I filled it with some anti-septic and plugged it with cotton wool. "Now I'll give her an anti-tetanus injection and we'd better get a good poultice on straight away. She's been brewing that abscess at the top of a seedy toe infection for some time. No wonder the poor old girl goes lame."

Sarah assured me that she and her sister would put the poultice on and bandage the foot up. However, I reasoned that, if I were to do it myself, it would prolong my visit and I might get a chance to know the family better. "Go and put the kettle on for some hot water for the poultice, and, while you are at it, make us a cup of tea. I am sure that David would like one," Mrs Clifton said, already questioning my motives, I believed.

"What a good idea," I replied. "I'll just inject the mare and then I'll come and help." I filled up the syringe and popped it into Merry's neck with Mrs Clifton holding her head.

"Do try and cheer Sarah up a bit. She's very depressed about not riding her horse."

I promised to do my best and walked off towards the kitchen door. Sarah called out for me to come in. She was busy taking a tray of cakes from the oven of a large Aga stove, on which the kettle was singing away.

"I've been told to cheer you up," I laughed. "It shouldn't be too difficult, because I hope we'll have Merry sound in two or three days. I'll have to get hold of your blacksmith and arrange for us to put a permanent dressing under the shoe."

Sarah brightened. "Are you sure?" she asked.

"Well, I can promise I'll pull out all the stops for you. Otherwise I know that you'll hide away with your books and I shan't see you again."

"Who on earth told you that?" She bridled. "That mother of mine says the most stupid things. Anyway what's wrong with reading?"

I hastily assured her that I was all in favour of books, and that I never had enough time to read as much as I would like. Further conversation was interrupted by the arrival of Ann and her mother.

"I hear you've found out what's wrong with Merry," Ann said, as she got the tea cups. "I said all along that that old Baker didn't know what he was doing." She obviously meant Charlie Baker, the blacksmith from the next village. It was hardly fair to blame him, because he would not notice a seedy toe when he was simply changing a shoe. When she confirmed it was Charlie, I said I would have a word with him and try to fix an appointment in about three days. I knew old Charlie well. He was a first-rate farrier, but his fondness for the Crown Inn tended to interfere with his activities. He looked after one of the local racing stables, where he was treated as one of the family. However they had often to send a van to winkle him out of his hostelry to get a horse plated for the races. One Christmas they had actually given him a small motor-bike in the hope that it might make him more available than he was on his old push-bike. This did not turn out as well as they had hoped. On New Year's Day, Charlie was emboldened to try one or two further-flung drinking haunts, with the result that he was found in a blackthorn bush, and the bike upside down against a large elm tree. Charlie, being in a somewhat relaxed state at the time, had suffered no injuries but the machine was never itself again.

Tea over, I went out and dressed the mare's foot. Finally leaving instructions for the next couple of days, and assuring the Cliftons that they only had to ring me if there were any problems with the mare, I drove off. I found Charlie Baker that evening in his usual seat by the dart board. At the cost of two pints, I got him to promise to meet me at the Cliftons', the following Friday afternoon at two o'clock.

When I told Billy what I had found in the horse's foot, he replied that if he had only been given some shoeing tools, he would no doubt have found the same thing. Anyhow he thanked me and said that he would call back on Friday to meet the blacksmith, as he knew I had a busy weekend ahead. I quickly answered that I would be easily able to fit in the visit, and that I had promised to meet Charlie there. Billy and Jim laughed, wondering whether it was really the blacksmith I had promised or one of the two girls that I was hurrying back to. I hotly denied their insinuations – but they remained firmly unconvinced.

I arrived promptly at two o'clock, to find that the girls were out in the jumping field. Joan Clifton was rushing about, raising the jumps and continually urging her daughters to 'hurry and jump'. Ann was riding her old jumper, and Sarah was on a big black horse of uncertain parentage. Ann jumped round the course without difficulty, and then Sarah turned her horse into the first fence. He resolutely refused to take any part in the entertainment, until Mrs Clifton approached from his rear brandishing a large branch out of an oak tree. He immediately set off with great gusto and proceeded to knock over all but two of the fences. Sarah got off with a determined look and told her mother to tie the top rail of the triple bar down tightly. Having supervised this operation, she remounted and then, to my horror, circled around to approach it from the wrong side. She stoked up the big horse, who took off in some amazement, hit the top hard and then sprawled on his belly through the two lower poles. Without giving him time to catch his breath, his rider aimed at the next fence. He stood back and cleared it by at least a foot, as he did all the remaining jumps. Sarah pulled up by me. "That'll teach the lazy devil," she laughed. "I've been wanting to do that for the last week."

"I hope you don't make a habit of living so dangerously." I ventured, picturing all my plans disintegrating with the demise of my newly-made acquaintance.

I enquired how Merry Queen was, and was told by her delighted owner that she was trotting sound on the grass. Mr Baker, she said, was up at the stables shoeing one of the other horses. I left her to follow with her horse and drove round to the house, gathered up my stuff and made my way to the mare's box. There was no sign of Charlie anywhere, although his tools were lying outside the tack room. I shouted his name in vain. The girls came into the yard, and suggested that he might have gone into the house. Ann put her horse away and went to search. I yelled his name again. Silence. Sarah began to look in the stables where the horse, which Charlie had been left to shoe, was as she had left it. I wandered up the row to the old cart stables, which were now used for the hens. I looked into the dark interior and could see nothing. Suddenly I heard a deep sigh. I pushed open the door and walked in. As my eyes became accustomed to the gloom I saw a figure up in the long hay rack and made out the dishevelled figure of Charlie, fast asleep, clutching a bottle half-full of beer. Gently I prised the bottle out of his hand, and unceremoniously tipped the remaining contents over his head. He woke with a start and looked at me with his bleary eyes. "What the devil are you playing at? Give me back my beer."

"Come on Charlie, you have had your beer and your kip. It's high time you started work again." Grumbling as he straightened his cramped limbs, he slowly prised himself out of his perch and dropped to the floor, put his cap back over his damp hair and reluctantly followed me out.

"Are you all right, Mr Baker?" Sarah asked when she saw his clothes smothered in hay.

"Don't worry. He's O.K. He must have been chasing a rat in your chicken house. Wasn't that it, Charlie?" I said, turning to my companion.

"That's it, Mr Dawson. Bloomin' great big 'un it was too." He picked up his tools as he passed them, and we went into Merry's stable. Sarah had removed the bandages, and I told Charlie to pick up its foot so that I could pack the cavity with some carbolic and chalk. I was halfway through the operation when Charlie started to sway. "I don't feel too good " he mumbled.

I shook his shoulder, "Wake up, for God's sake. You're not going to rest until we've got this foot finished and shod." Hastily I finished packing in the cement and told the sleepy farrier to bang on the shoe. He had filed down the last clinch and put down her foot, when he coughed apologetically. "I think I'll just go and have a sit-down, Miss." And went off into the tack room.

Sarah pulled the mare out and, to my relief, she trotted as soundly as the proverbial bell. "I must get her saddle and take her for a proper exercise," she said, and made to go up the yard.

"Hold on a minute," I cried, "I might not see you again for months unless you get another lame horse. How about coming out to the cinema and a meal this weekend?"

She seemed surprised by my invitation, but she agreed. I arranged a time for Saturday and left happily for my car.

"David," she called. "Mr Baker's asleep on the corn bin. Do you think he'll be safe there?"

"Don't worry," I grinned." He won't move for some time and he can't hurt himself in the corn."

"Good-bye then." She paused. "And thanks for the invitation."

As I drove off, I was feeling extremely pleased with myself. I had cured the horse and made a start on what I had the feeling was going to be a most rewarding affair. Charlie slept until seven o'clock, when he climbed onto his push-bike and pedalled off without a word. Sarah had told her mother that I had asked her out to dinner, and her mother had winked knowingly.

## MARRIAGE – HUMAN STYLE

FOLLOWING my first visit to the Clifton's farm, I began to make more frequent journeys up to the red house on the Ridgeway. Under the thinly veiled pretext of looking at some minor ailment in one of the horses, I took to dropping in most evenings. Even the attempts of the girls to turn me into a show-jump rider failed to discourage me. I think that I unwittingly served as light relief from the hard work of their day as I tried in vain to master the skills of precision jumping. Either the horse or I would lose patience and set sail at one of the obstacles only to begin a demolition job on their practice jumping course. However, they say that love is blind, and Sarah did not seem to be put off by my amateur efforts. As the summer progressed, we grew closer and the outcome must have been obvious to everyone but ourselves. So it was with considerable surprise that I found myself stopping the car one evening and suggesting that it would save a lot of petrol and excuses if we were to get married. Sarah was speechless, which did little for my morale, and neither of us could do justice to a particularly fine baked alaska that a friend produced for our dinner. For three days I was kept in suspense, until she casually remarked to me as I was rebuilding yet another practice fence that she thought it would save a lot of timber if she were to accept my offer.

By the time that our engagement was officially announced, the hunting season was in full swing. One of the spin-offs from my new attachment to the Clifton family was that I was allowed to hunt their horses. The difference between riding a well-schooled show-jumper or event horse and scrubbing round on a retired 'chaser was comparable to driving a Rolls Royce after having struggled along in a 'souped up' old M.G., which had developed a tendency to asthma. The novel feeling of confidence that you would actually negotiate every fence you attempted was exhilarating.

Both Sarah and Ann hunted, the latter going like a rocket, always egging me on to tackle some more horrifying ditch or fence than the last. Luckily for me, it was such a very wet winter, that my glasses were constantly awash with rain. It was amazing how brave I could be when I was virtually blind. Sarah was hunting a young bay horse called Patrick, which she was bringing on for the next year's one-day events. Her idea of education for Patrick was the embodiment of patience – so much so that we teased her that she was overtiring him if she actually allowed him to gallop over more than one ploughed field. However she had the last laugh on us in that she used to bring him home quite unscathed every time, whereas our mounts were plastered with mud and pricked like pin-cushions with thorns. Ann and I would spend an hour probing our horses' legs and dabbing on antiseptic, while Sarah had done up her precious steed and was already languishing in a hot bath.

Patrick had been bought about three months before for a ridiculously low price from my old friend Peter Davey. It was to worry him for the rest of his life that he had slipped up in not recognising the potential of the rather plain gelding he had palmed off onto Mrs Clifton. Not only did the ugly duckling win many contests as a jumper, but he was in the top flight of ladies' show hunters for several seasons. It is fair to say that Peter recouped his losses over the next few years by doubling the asking price for anything that the Cliftons tried to buy off him.

Peter Davey was a horse dealer of the old school. He had a yard near Kingsclere on the Hampshire border, and turned out a constant succession of ponies and horses. I was a frequent visitor, because he would never sell a horse without my examination. Since half his purchases were far from sound, I had a running battle with him, trying to discover the particular catch in any deal. His father had been a dealer before him and he knew all the tricks used to disguise a horse's shortcomings. Such simple ploys as trotting up a horse as fast as possible, and so disguising chronic minor lameness, were chicken-feed to Peter. He had a steady flow of patter to distract one from concentrating on examining a horse. He would fuss about a tiny bump on a fore limb and ask continual questions about it, hoping to divert my attention from the large bony spavin on one of its hocks. On one occasion his attempt at hiding a case of laryngeal paralysis in a big hunter misfired badly. As I walked to the box with him, a bottle crashed to the ground and broke into a thousand pieces. By the time we had covered the last few yards, the horse had trodden on a splinter of glass and cut his foot. His son emerged from the stable to be soundly abused by the dealer for his incompetence. Peter said that he had instructed him to wash the horse's mouth out, so that it was clean for me to examine. This was so unlikely a tale that I felt I had to investigate the truth. Sending Peter out to get some hot water, I dabbed my finger in the pool of fluid which was still on the floor and immediately recognised the smell and feel of glycerine. So that was what the old devil had been trying! There was a popularly held belief that half a pint of glycerine put into the back of the horse's throat would mask the noise of a "roarer" for a short time. I said nothing to Peter, but, when I returned a week later to examine the horse, I made sure that it had a few mouthfuls of grass before we worked him and thus cleared his throat of the lubricant. That one did NOT pass!

Like all dealers of his kind, Peter would go to any lengths to earn an extra couple of pounds. One morning when I was called to see a horse with colic, he was busy in the yard trying to sell a lady a second-hand hunting crop. He was asking five pounds and the customer was sticking at three. I treated the horse and left his son to keep an eye on him. Returning at lunch-time to see my patient, I was astounded to find Peter and his lady customer still bartering over the wretched crop. He had taken her into his sitting room and, with the aid of several strong gin and tonics had got her up to four quid. Finally, to his obvious delight, the deal was completed at four pounds and five shillings. While I was sitting down to lunch with the family, there was a knock at the door, and a retired trainer came in. I knew that he was more than a little down on his luck, and I had a shrewd idea as to the reason for his visit. They withdraw to the office, and, when they emerged in a couple of minutes, the ex-trainer was stuffing a roll of notes into his pocket. Later, when his wife asked how much he had given him, Peter replied somewhat shame-facedly that he had let him have two hundred pounds.

"How on earth can you spend all morning trying to screw a paltry pound for an old crop that you picked up at a sale for a few shillings, and then hand out that much money, which you know you'll never see again?"

Peter laughed, "You'll never understand that, David. You're either born a dealer or you aren't and, if not, you'll never appreciate the thrill of winning a contest of minds. You can't understand the wonderful feeling in selling someone a horse, when all they called into the yard for was a hundred-weight of potatoes. By the way," he went on, "your bill for last month was far too big. I'm not one of your rich racehorse clients you know."

I knew what was coming. Every month we had the same battle. He would collect an old ledger from the office. This had once belonged to one of his uncles, who had been the local vet. He would point to an item such as *Attention to horse's teeth, three shillings and six pence.* "There now, he would say. "Three and six, and you've got the affrontery to charge me ten shillings."

I would patiently turn to the front of the ledger yet again and point out the date, which read *July 1869.* Reasoning that he could have sold me a horse then for some five pounds, whereas today he would want at least two hundred, I would alter my monthly account from, say, fourteen pounds to five hundred and sixty pounds. This usually had the prompt effect of causing him to reach for his cheque book and pay my fee without further argument.

The arrangements for our wedding occasionally briefly occupied the Clifton family. The main problem was to find a date that did not clash with some horse show. This was far from easy, since they attended at least two shows a week from March to October, and it seemed they were all equally important. Somebody hopefully suggested that we could delay the decision until one of the horses went lame, so that they would have to miss at least one competition. Sarah was not struck by this casual approach and acidly pointed out that if we were to fall in with the idea, presumably I would be expected to return from my honeymoon to treat the unfortunate animal.

The final decision was prompted by my new dog. I had recently come by an English setter of high pedigree, but low habits. His house-training had been sadly neglected by his breeders, to the extent that he still did not realise the propriety of relieving himself in decent privacy. I called in at the farm one evening and found the family in the jumping field where they were trying a new pony over the fences. My mother-in-law-to-be was as usual bustling about the field, urging her daughters to greater feats with the pony. Dressed in her customary working clothes with the addition of a large pair of her husband's wellington boots, she was finally satisfied with the course and stood back to see the pony perform. Meanwhile, my dog, having investigated the various jumps, wandered up to Joan, sniffed around her, casually lifted his leg and filled up the interior of her left boot. Horror-struck, I watched this performance from the far side of the field. However, so engrossed was the occupant of the boot, that she never noticed the assault. The jumping over, Mrs Clifton started off for the house. "Really Jack," she said crossly to her husband, "why can't you look after your boots properly? One of them's got a hole in it and has let the water through."

Jack had also apparently been watching my hound, who had by now gone off to look for a rabbit in the hedge. He burst out laughing. "Don't blame my boots. That was that bloody dog of David's. Though it's a bit hard that he should have mistaken you for a tree stump!"

"Well that settles it," Joan answered. "We must get these

157

two married, if only to keep that wretched dog away from the farm."

So the great day was planned for the end of April. Reluctantly it was conceded that they would take only one horse to the Oxford Show, so that Ann could be back in time for the wedding after lunch. This meant that Sarah was left to feed all the calves and the other ponies on her wedding morning – a grudge, together with my having to dash off on a colic case half an hour after the birth of our first child a year later, which has never been forgotten or forgiven. Two days before the wedding, nothing had been arranged. However, a sudden last minute surge of panic brought into being a marquee, clothes for the bride and bridesmaid, drink and a super two-tiered wedding cake, decorated with a sugar show-jumper and racehorse, forelegs intertwined. Alas, the temptation was too much for Bugsby, my trusty dog, who stole into the larder and removed the top tier on the night before the wedding. There is no doubt that this act of blatant vandalism finally cleared any doubts which my mother-in-law might have had about going through with the wedding.

Sarah, like the other members of her family, had not been a regular church-goer. Indeed it is fair to say that her entry up the aisle of the little Norman church in the village was her first sight of the interior of any English church. She had visited various cathedrals in France and Spain, when taken on a whirlwind tour of the continent by some relations, trying to cure their daughter of some unsuitable romance. However, the mysteries of the service were a closed book to her. This is not to say that I was a regular member of the congregation. But one of the major results of a public school education is some knowledge of church services, so as I stood by my best man at the front of the church, I was at least reasonably in control of my senses.

The vicar was a kindly old man, who unfortunately suffered from lapses during which he thought he was the re-incarnation of St John the Divine. To cure him of these flights of fancy, he was regularly removed to a nearby church rest home. Unknown to me, he had returned from such a visit only two days before our wedding. The effect of being disillusioned from his saintly imaginings had caused such considerable mental shock, that it was difficult to tell whether he or my bride was the more nervous. Their prayer books wavered like branches of a tree in a strong gale, and their voices croaked like the famous Aristophanes' frogs. Somehow we got through the service, despite a loud guffaw from my newly acquired father-in-law who was overcome by the sight of a very large hole in the sole of one of my best wedding shoes. He nudged his wife and asked in a loud stage whisper whether David really could afford to keep their daughter, as he clearly could not afford to pay the cobbler.

The service ended without further mishap, except for an altercation between my god-daughter and Sarah as to which way they turned on leaving the altar. This would not have mattered too much except that the little girl was firmly clutching the end of the train. The tug-of-war which ensued did little for the arrangement of Sarah's hair and head-dress. The photographs, subseqently taken outside the church, gave rise to many queries from our friends as to what had really been going on between us in the vestry!

The reception was, as far as I can remember, a success. It was marred only by the interminable length of my speech, which, at the time, I had thought to be both brief and witty. Alas, the best man was unkind enough to record the festivities on cine film which emphasises only too clearly the preference of the guests for the refreshments rather than for my carefully chosen phrases. Still, I hope that it has served to turn my own children's thoughts toward the Registry Office rather than risk a full-blown wedding themselves.

Our departure from the party was speeded by Joan Clifton's sudden desire for Sarah to bring out her show-hack, so she could put it through its paces for my sister who had expressed a polite interest in the horses – an interest, I may say, that was never more than a fleeting one, since she lived in the art world in Chelsea and regarded all four-legged creatures as dirty and dangerous. Deciding that it was better to nip that particular idea in the bud, before my family's total ignorance on all matters equine was cruelly exposed, I grabbed hold of my wife and set off for our honeymoon, which was, I suspect, about as successful as most ventures of its kind. We spent three weeks in Majorca getting to know each other and trying to hide our true characters from each other for as long as we decently could.

Apart from the usual traumas to which honeymoons are heir, ours was memorable for some execrable hotel food, which tended to find its way down the throat of a permanently hungry donkey, who lived at the end of a seemingly endless moped ride along a cliff top. This was particularly exciting in that neither Sarah nor I had ever ventured on such a machine. Perilously we explored the island from the enforced imprisonment of the tram-lines, into which I managed unerringly to steer the front wheel. On one occasion we followed some tourists to a shabby Flamenco display, which was compered for our doubtful benefit by a Yorkshireman giving a poor man's imitation of Wilfred Pickles. At last it was with some feelings of relief that we boarded our primitive Dakota to fly to home and work.

Our arrival at our new house, built by an old friend, Keith Piggott, and the birth place of his well-known son, Lester, was to be the high point of my new life. Poised to carry my wife over the threshold I discovered to my horror that the keys were nowhere to be found. So Sarah was ignominiously shoved through the kitchen window which I had to break to facilitate her entry. But we had not realised that the kitchen door was locked from the outside and, after extricating my beloved through the same window, I had to repeat the manoeuvre through an upstairs landing window. Once having forced possession of our home, we celebrated our arrival with tea in a wine glass, sitting on two packing cases left behind by the last occupant.

It was hardly an auspicious beginning. But, at least, we confronted each other with the thought that things could only improve. As indeed they certainly have, because ours is surely one of those marriages that could be labelled "Made in Heaven".